The Difficult
Cesarean Delivery

Safeguards and Pitfalls

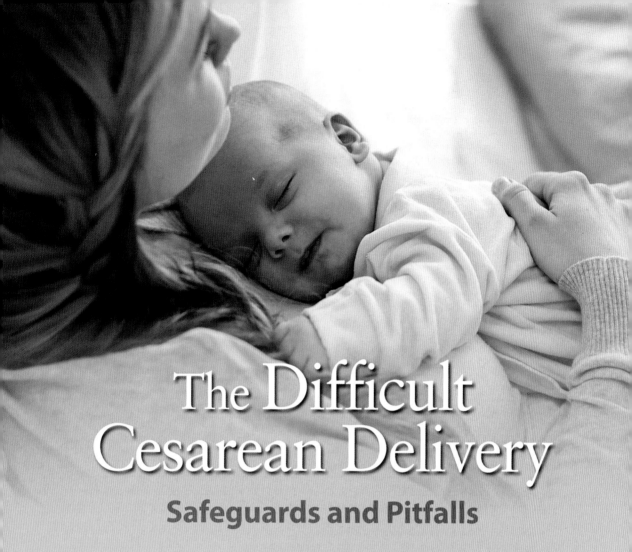

The Difficult Cesarean Delivery

Safeguards and Pitfalls

Guy I. Benrubi, MD
Emeritus Chair
Robert J. Thompson
  Professor
Division of Gynecologic
  Oncology
Department of Obstetrics
  and Gynecology
University of Florida College
  of Medicine
Jacksonville, Florida

Erin H. Burnett, MD
Assistant Professor
Chief, Division of Maternal
  Fetal Medicine
Program Director of
  Ultrasound and Prenatal
  Diagnosis
Clerkship Director
Department of Obstetrics
  and Gynecology
University of Florida College
  of Medicine
Jacksonville, Florida

Kristy K. Ward, MD, MAS
Gynecologic Oncologist
Texas Oncology
Houston, Texas

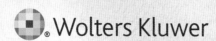

. Wolters Kluwer

Philadelphia • Baltimore • New York • London
Buenos Aires • Hong Kong • Sydney • Tokyo

Acquisitions Editor: Chris Teja
Development Editor: Carole Wonsiewicz
Editorial Coordinator: Tim Rinehart
Marketing Manager: Phyllis Hitner
Production Project Manager: Barton Dudlick
Design Coordinator: Stephen Druding
Manufacturing Coordinator: Beth Welsh
Prepress Vendor: TNQ Technologies

9 8 7 6 5 4 3 2 1

Printed in China

Library of Congress Cataloging-in-Publication Data

ISBN-13: 978-1-975116-67-5

Cataloging in Publication data available on request from publisher.

shop.lww.com

To Rob, LGs, Darian, Freddie, Poonch, and Fidelica

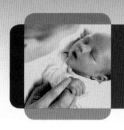

CONTENTS

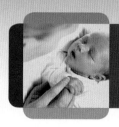

CONTRIBUTORS

C. David Adair, MD
Professor and Vice Chair
Division Director of Maternal Fetal
  Medicine
Department of Obstetrics and Gynecology
University of Tennessee College of Medicine
Chattanooga, Tennessee

Anjum Anwar, MD, FCPS
Anesthesia Patient Safety Fellow,
Department of Anesthesia,
University of Florida College of Medicine,
Jacksonville, Florida

Ted Bangert, MD
Obstetric Anesthesia Fellow
Department of Anesthesia
University of Florida College of Medicine
Jacksonville, Florida

Guy I. Benrubi, MD
Emeritus Chair
Robert J. Thompson Professor
Division of Gynecologic Oncology
Department of Obstetrics and Gynecology
University of Florida College of Medicine
Jacksonville, Florida

Todd Boren, MD
Associate Professor
Division of Gynecologic Oncology
Department of Obstetrics and Gynecology
University of Tennessee College of Medicine
Chattanooga, Tennessee

Sarah Boyd, MD
Department of Obstetrics and Gynecology
University of Tennessee College of Medicine
Chattanooga, Tennessee

Erin H. Burnett, MD
Assistant Professor
Chief, Division of Maternal Fetal Medicine
Program Director of Ultrasound and
  Prenatal Diagnosis
Clerkship Director
Department of Obstetrics and Gynecology
University of Florida College of Medicine
Jacksonville, Florida

Shae Connor, MD
Associate Professor
Department of Obstetrics and Gynecology
University of Tennessee College of Medicine
Chattanooga, Tennessee

Stephen DePasquale, MD
Chair, Department of Obstetrics and
  Gynecology
Associate Professor and Co-Director
  Research
Department of Obstetrics and Gynecology
University of Tennessee College of Medicine
Chattanooga, Tennessee

S. Kyle Gonzales, MD
Associate Professor
Division of Maternal Fetal Medicine
University of Tennessee College of Medicine
Chattanooga, Tennessee

Joanna Kee-Sampson, MD
Assistant Professor
Department of Vascular and Interventional
  Radiology
University of Florida College of Medicine
Jacksonville, Florida

Travis E. Meyer, MD
Assistant Professor
Department of Vascular and Interventional
    Radiology
University of Florida College of Medicine
Jacksonville, Florida

Tripp Nelson, MD
Assistant Professor
Division of Maternal Fetal Medicine
Department of Obstetrics and Gynecology
University of Tennessee College of Medicine
Chattanooga, Tennessee

Daniel Siragusa, MD
Professor and Chief, Division of Vascular
    and Interventional Radiology
Program Director, Vascular and
    Interventional Radiology Fellowship
Program Director, Interventional Radiology-
    Integrated Residency
Department of Interventional Radiology
University of Florida College of Medicine
Jacksonville, Florida

Kristen Vanderhoef, MD
Assistant Professor
Department of Anesthesia
University of Florida College of Medicine
Jacksonville, Florida

Kimberly Vickers, RDMS
Lead Sonographer Prenatal Diagnostics
    Program
Department of Obstetrics and Gynecology
UF Health Jacksonville
Jacksonville, Florida

Kristy K. Ward, MD, MAS
Gynecologic Oncologist
Texas Oncology
Houston, Texas

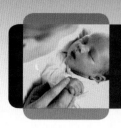

PREFACE

Cesarean delivery is the most commonly performed surgical procedure in the United States, with the exception of cataract removal. It is the first major surgical procedure that is mastered by trainees during residency in obstetrics and gynecology. Depending on scope of practice, a generalist obstetrician and gynecologist will feel most confident performing this procedure compared to any other consistently performed during her/his career. One of the consequent problems, however, is that "familiarity breeds contempt." In the vast majority of Cesarean section situations, the outcome for the mother, baby, and surgeon is usually happy and reassuring. Unfortunately *difficult* Cesarean sections are being encountered with increasing frequency and not infrequently with unhappy and disastrous results. The two most common causes for the difficult Cesarean are (1) the obesity epidemic and (2) the increasing occurrence of placenta accreta spectrum (PAS). The latter is a consequence of the high Cesarean section rate in the United States and the world and the consequent number of repeat Cesarean deliveries.

This book addresses the most common challenges of the *difficult* Cesarean section and presents strategies to avoid potential pitfalls. Several chapters approach the same problem from different author's perspective. It is the editors' belief that multiplicity of views enhances understanding of physiology and pathology and thus leads to optimal management. The editors would like to thank all authors for their contributions and the sharing of their expertise.

The editors would also like to thank Chris Teja of Wolters Kluwer who was instrumental in the conception and decision to proceed with this project, Tim Rinehart of Wolters Kluwer for his technical support and incredible patience, and Carole Wonsiewicz who provided invaluable editing, without which this project could not be completed. A great "thank you" is due to Marsha Cole—without her expertise, perseverance, and selfless devotion, this book could not have been written.

*"…Don't put off things till it's too late.
You are the DJ of your fate."*

—Vikram Seth (The Golden Gate, 1986)

"Raccomode tes vetements tu les porteras 100 ans" (mend your garments and you will wear them for 100 years). Old European proverb; interpretation: nothing should be neglected.

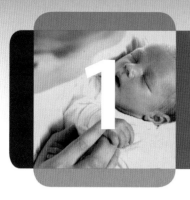

The Impact of Cesarean Delivery on Maternal Mortality and Morbidity

Guy I. Benrubi

How a society treats its female population reflects the quality of life in that society. One can assess the overall human condition of a society by the amount of resources dedicated to the well-being, education, and equal civil status of women. Maternal mortality statistics are one of the most direct indicators of the importance governmental and nongovernmental institutions direct toward the well-being of women. Birth is in the most direct interest of a society. Ensuring safe pregnancy and safe birth should be a priority to the safety and protection of its citizenry just as important as internal law and order, border integrity, and disaster protection and response.

One of the measures of "development" worldwide during the 20th and 21st centuries is a consistent and sharp drop in maternal mortality. The drop does not only indicate a medial delivery system that is technologically advanced but also points to the educational, nutritional, and equality achievements in the entity. In Europe and other developed countries during the last 150 years, there has been remarkable progress in the reduction of maternal mortality, yet this goal has not been achieved in the United States.[1,2] *Maternal mortality* is measured by the pregnancy-related mortality ratio, further defined as the number of deaths of pregnant women that are due to a pregnancy complication. The most recent Centers for Disease Control and Prevention (CDC, 2014) report on the current status in the United States is as follows:

"Since the Pregnancy Mortality Surveillance System was implemented, the number of reported pregnancy-related deaths in the United States steadily increased from 7.2 deaths per 100,000 live births in 1987 to 18.0 deaths per 100,000 live births in 2014. The graph below shows trends in pregnancy-related mortality ratios defined as the number of pregnancy-related deaths per 100,000 live births in the United States between 1987 and 2014 (the latest available year of data)."[1] (Figure 1-1).

This rise in maternal deaths is magnified by the estimate that approximately 50% of maternal deaths in the United States are preventable.

This question of why in the United States there is such a dramatic increase in the pregnancy-related mortality ratio coupled with the dramatic increase in both technological advances and understanding of pregnancy physiology is puzzling and many are searching for answers. Several authors suggest the following factors[3-8]:

1. *Inconsistency of level of obstetric care in areas of the United States* with many sophisticated settings with the latest equipment and most experience practitioners versus other settings where births occur in primitive conditions. Very frequently deteriorating clinical conditions are identified too late. There is a lack of a standard approach mandated either by professional self-regulation or legislative statute.[3-5]

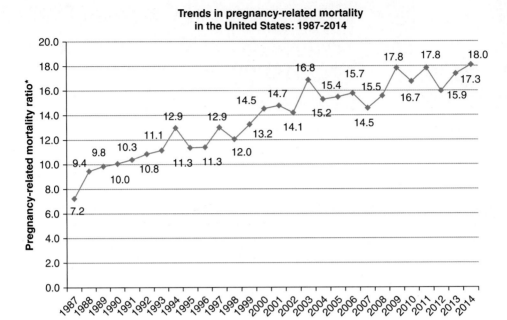

Note: Number of pregnancy-related deaths per 100,000 live births per year.

FIGURE 1-1 Trends in pregnancy-related mortality in the United States: 1987-2014. (Reprinted from CDC: Pregnancy Mortality Surveillance Systems. Accessed 1/2019. https://www.cdc.gov/reproductivehealth/maternalinfanthealth/pregnancy-mortality-surveillance-system.htm.)

2. *The increasing percentage of pregnant patients with chronic health conditions without access to affordable prenatal care.* Hypertension, diabetes, and particularly obesity are on the increase. In the United States, uninsured patients are three to four times more likely to die from maternal complications than insured women. The most effective solution is a healthcare system that provides affordable prenatal care to all pregnant patients. Several states have addressed this problem by expanding Medicaid eligibility to pregnant patients, but there are huge gaps.[4,5]

3. *A lack of good and accurate data* which can lead to stronger analysis of the causes for each maternal death and provide a basis for evidence-based interventions. There is no national forum where data and best practices from all states can be reviewed. Only about half of states have established maternal mortality review committees, such as Florida's Pregnancy Associated Mortality Review (PAMR) committee and the Florida Perinatal Quality Cooperative.[3,4]

4. *Reporting inconsistencies.* There has always been concern that births either at home or at birthing centers run by "lay" midwives are underreported including the complications encountered in those settings. Many states lack legislative mandates to report all maternal complications regardless of site of service, not just in hospitals. For example, it was just in 2018 that the state of Florida passed such a statute and many states do not currently have equivalent legislation.

5. *There are huge healthcare disparities and statistics in certain populations in the United States.* The following maternal/mortality statistics per 100,000 births demonstrate this: white women is 12.4, for African-Americans 40.0, and for

Hispanic and other nonwhites 17.8. The ratio has increased across all populations, even in white women an increase of 7 to 12.4 during the last 20 years.[5-8]

Worldwide the main cause of maternal mortality is hemorrhage.[6] From the CDC statistics (2011-2014), the causes of maternal mortality in the United States were attributed to approximately 25% from cardiovascular disease and cardiomyopathy, 12.8% from infections and sepsis, and hypertensive disorders (6.8%).[1] However, latest estimates for the United States show hemorrhage now is the leading cause of maternal death.[3] Statistics from Florida in 2018 implicate hemorrhage as the cause of death in 20.7% of cases and hypertension and cardiomyopathy each accounted for 13.8%.[9]

These discouraging results showed that 55.3% of these deaths were deemed preventable, and in another 18.4% of the deaths "there was a possible chance to alter the outcome."[9] The conclusion is that in almost 75% of the maternal deaths in Florida, the standard of care was not met.

The other salient statistic is that 76.2% of these deaths occurred during or after a cesarean delivery.[9] It was not possible to glean from the data what percentage was associated with complicated cesarean deliveries. However, it is reasonable to expect that patients who were obese, had abnormal placentation such as accreta or percreta, or had previous multiple cesarean sections accounted for the majority of these deaths. A list of maternal conditions which lead to complications during and after a cesarean delivery include[11]:

1. Grand multiparity
2. Placenta previa
3. Placenta accreta
4. Repeat cesarean section (especially after three previous sections)
5. Morbidly obese patient
6. Fetal anomalies
7. Transverse fetal lie
8. Maternal coagulopathy
9. Large uterine fibroids
10. Maternal problems leading to anesthesia hazards
11. Multiple gestation

Despite the discouraging statistics indicating that at least half of these deaths might have been prevented if emergency procedures were in place, the encouraging news is that the PAMR identified the causes of these deaths and recommended preventive measures. These recommendations are being disseminated to all obstetric providers and hospitals in the state via multiple venues. The following are the PAMR committee recommendations. These as well as others will be discussed in greater detail in the chapters of this book.[10]

Florida Pregnancy Mortality Review (PAMR) findings:

1. Hospitals establish a process for recognizing and responding immediately when a patient's condition appears to be worsening
2. Hospitals develop written criteria which describe early warning signs of a change/deterioration in a patient's condition and when to seek further assistance
3. Always discuss with patient and family the possibilities and need for transfer
4. If placental disorder is suspected, immediately request a Maternal-Fetal Medicine consultation

5. Imaging modalities/results are not always perfect. Regardless of imaging results, if you suspect problem, transfer to tertiary facility
6. Staff is aware of potential high risk for accreta: cesarean section, placenta previa, multiparity, myomectomy, repetitive curettage, and advanced maternal age
7. A low-lying anterior placenta could be an ominous sign in patient with multiple prior cesarean sections
8. Consider early transfer to tertiary center for access to sufficient blood supply and subspecialists
9. Implement a hemorrhage protocol including massive transfusion protocol, simulation drills, and hemorrhage cart
10. Alert blood bank for potential massive transfusion
11. Alert anesthesia
12. Establish availability of expert surgical and medical teams
13. Familiarity with aortic compression and other temporizing methods

The critical aspect of all of these recommendations is the understanding that the *difficult cesarean section* is a different surgical and medical entity when compared to the *routine cesarean delivery*. Providers caring for such patients must be prepared to ask for and receive appropriate additional support in order to avoid catastrophe. The hope of the authors of this book is to present essential and practical information and procedures which can help implement proper standards of care and reduce those statistics regarding possible preventable maternal deaths.

REFERENCES

1. Pregnancy Mortality Surveillance Systems. Available at https://www.cdc.gov/reproductivehealth/maternalinfanthealth/pregnancy-mortality-surveillance-system.htm. Accessed 1/2019.
2. Trends in Maternal Mortality: 1990 to 2013. *Estimates by WHO, UNICEF, UNFPA, The World Bank and the United Nations Population Division.* Geneva: World Health Organization; 2014. Available at http://www.who.int/reproductivehealth/publications/monitoring/maternal-mortality-2013/en/. [cited 2014 Jul 18].
3. Pregnancy-Associated Mortality Review. Florida Department of Health, Division of Community Health Promotion. Pregnancy-Related Deaths Due to Hemorrhage, 1999-2012. Available at http://www.floridahealth.gov/statistics-and-data/PAMR/_documents/Pregnancy-Related%20Deaths%20Due%20to%20Hemorrhage,%201999–2012%20Brief.pdf. Accessed 1/19.
4. Agrawal P. Maternal mortality and morbidity in the United States of America. *Bull World Health Organ.* 2015;93(3):135.
5. Carroll A. Why is US maternal mortality rising? *J Am Med Assoc.* 2017;318(4):321. https://jamanetwork.com/journals/jama/fullarticle/2645089/.
6. Lu M. Reducing maternal mortality in the United States. *J Am Med Assoc.* 2018;320(12):1237-1238.
7. Berg CS, Callaghan WM, Syverson C, Henderson Z. Pregnancy related mortality in the United States 1998 to 2005. *Obstet Gynecol.* 2010;116(6):1302-1309.
8. ACOG Practice Bulletin Number 183; October 2017.
9. Obstetric Hemorrhage Initiative. Florida Perinatal Quality Cooperative. 2018. Available at www.health.usf.edu/publichealth/chiles/fpqc/OHI.htm. Accessed February 1, 2019.
10. Committee on Maternal Mortality and Morbidity ACOG District XII Message to Providers and Message to Hospitals, 2018. Available at http://www.floridahealth.gov/statistics-and-data/PAMR/. Accessed February 1, 2019.
11. World Health Organization. Available at https://www.who.int/news-room/fact-sheets/detail/maternal-mortality. Accessed 1/2019.

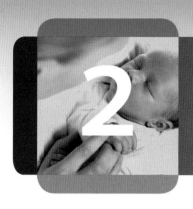

2

The Obesity Epidemic

Guy I. Benrubi

Obesity and unwanted weight gain are now recognized as a spectrum of a chronic or noncommunicable disease.[1-4] Unwanted weight gain leading to overweight and obesity has become a main driver of the global rise in noncommunicable diseases. Comorbidities such as type 2 diabetes mellitus, hypertension, and cardiovascular disease exact a heavy toll on overweight and obese individuals.[5] Additionally, psychological and social effects on overweight individuals make them vulnerable to discrimination in their personal and work lives, in addition to low self-esteem and depression.[6] All of these factors contribute to huge healthcare costs and loss of productivity as well as decreased life expectancy.

The effect of obesity on life expectancy, both on the individual and on society, frequently is underappreciated. An article in the *Wall Street Journal* (2018) brought this effect to the attention of the public. The article pointed out that despite total cost of health care and despite technological advances at the highest level, the United States trails other developed nations in life expectancy.[7] The recent Global BMI Collaboration reported that obese populations have higher mortality regardless of country. Furthermore, according to the Organization for Economic Cooperation and Development (OECD) Health Statistics 2018, 40% of the US population is obese, as opposed to 17% in France, 13% in Sweden, and 4.2% in Japan, the country with the highest life expectancy.[8]

Obesity results from an interaction between a genetic predisposition to weight gain and environmental influences. Thus, there are very pronounced differences in the prevalence rates of obesity and being overweight among different populations. As will be seen below, the prevalence of obesity occurs highest in those populations most likely to present for health care at safety-net hospitals.[9]

The most accurate measures of body fat, such as underwater weighing, dual-energy x-ray absorptiometry (DEXA) scanning, computed tomography (CT), and magnetic resonance imaging (MRI), are impractical and expensive for use in most clinical encounters. Estimates of body fat, such as body mass index (BMI, calculated by dividing the body weight in kilograms by height in meters squared, or kg/m^2) and waist circumference, have limitations but are easily obtained and sufficient in most situations.

Body mass index allows comparison of weights independently of stature across populations. However, it should be remembered that in certain populations, such as body builders, the standard definitions do not apply. Also, certain populations may have different thresholds for concerning BMI. In South Asians, for instance, evidence suggests that BMI-adjusted percent body fat is greater than other populations.[10]

In 1998, the National Institutes of Health (NIH) Expert Panel on the Identification, Evaluation, and Treatment of Overweight and Obesity in Adults adopted the World Health Organization (WHO) classification for overweight and obesity. The WHO classification, which predominantly applied to people of European ancestry, assigns increasing risk for comorbid conditions, including hypertension, type 2 diabetes mellitus, and cardiovascular disease—to persons with a higher BMI relative to persons of normal weight (BMI of 18.5-25 kg/m^2). Thus it defines a BMI of 25 to 29 as overweight, a BMI of 30 as obese, and a BMI of 40 as extremely obese.[11]

What is even more concerning is that the prevalence of obesity seems to be increasing in the United States and in the world. In 2001, the Surgeon General issued a "Call to Action" on the obesity problem, but the call drew a minimal response from the responsible federal agencies, and Americans continued to consume an average of 3800 calories per person per day or about twice the daily requirement.[12]

In the most recently published United States report (2015-2016), almost 40% of adults in this country are at a BMI $\geq$ 30 kg/m^2 and almost 20% of youth are obese.[13]

These increases represent a tripling in obesity prevalence rates of the US population since the 1960s. Interestingly, during this time, the prevalence of overweight (BMI $\geq$ 25 and <30 kg/m^2) has remained stable in both men and women while that of extreme obesity (BMI $\geq$ 40 kg/m^2) has undergone a ninefold increase from 0.9% in 1960 to 1962 to 8.1% in 2017. Thus currently only $\sim$ 30% of the US population is considered to have a healthy weight (BMI between 18.5 and 25 kg/m^2).[14]

Increases in weight and obesity tend to peak between the ages of 40 and 60 years. But additional demographic studies show that women, as well as men, who did not attend college have higher rates. Women also had higher rates in those groups with lower incomes.[9]

The rise in obesity prevalence rates has disproportionately affected US minority populations. The highest prevalence rates of obesity by race and ethnicity are currently reported in blacks, native Americans, and Hispanics, reaching obesity prevalence rates of 50% and higher for Hispanic and black women.[9]

The problem is not limited to the United States. Historically, international obesity rates had been lower, and most developing countries considered undernutrition to be a bigger priority. However, international rates of overweight and obesity have been rising steadily for the past several decades and, in many countries, are now meeting or exceeding those of the United States. Between 1975 and 2016, worldwide, the number of adults with obesity increased over sixfold.[15] The rise in obesity rates is expected to continue for decades, as current obese adolescents mature into adults. This growth in the worldwide prevalence of overweight and obesity is thought to be primarily driven by economic and technological advancements in all developing societies. In growing economies, there is more time spent in sedentary work and less in manual labor. Additionally, dietary changes with increasing total calories and more processed foods have enhanced this phenomenon. The implications of this to healthcare providers dealing with immigrant populations are that unlike previous decades where the effects of malnutrition had to be addressed, now the effects of obesity have become paramount.

POTENTIAL COMPLICATIONS OF OBESITY IN PREGNANCY

Obesity can have a dramatic and often catastrophic impact on pregnancy outcome. Obesity in pregnancy has been associated with poor perinatal and neonatal outcomes.[16] Obese mothers have an increased risk of pregnancy complications such as anemia, hypertension, preeclampsia, preterm delivery, emergency cesarean section, and gestational diabetes. Though emergency cesarean rates vary so widely that comparisons are almost meaningless, reportedly in morbidly obese women, the cesarean delivery is significantly increased, and in some studies, by severalfold. It stands to reason, and it has been documented, that surgery in the morbidly obese patient poses many surgical, anesthetic, and logistical difficulties.[16]

Obesity is considered a major and frequent risk factor for developing complications in pregnancy. The incidence of pulmonary embolism and primary postpartum hemorrhage is increased. Anesthesia-related complications are frequent. Neonatal consequences of obesity include an increased rate of congenital anomalies, stillbirths, and macrosomia, and somewhat less frequently shoulder dystocia.[17]

There is an increased risk of spontaneous abortion and recurrent miscarriage. Obese women are also at an increased risk of delivering infants with neural tube defects; hydrocephaly; and cardiovascular, orofacial, and limb reduction anomalies. Obese gravidas are 40% more likely to experience stillbirth compared with nonobese gravidas. Antinatally, compared with normal-weight women, obese women are at an increased risk of cardiac dysfunction, proteinuria, sleep apnea, nonalcoholic fatty liver disease, gestational diabetes mellitus, and preeclampsia. There is an increase incidence of postpartum endometritis in both spontaneously delivered as well as those obese women delivered by cesarean section.[18]

In one study, the median duration of labor from 4 to 10 cm of cervical dilation was significantly longer in overweight and obese women.[19] Allowing a longer first stage of labor before performing cesarean delivery for labor arrest should be considered in obese women. An inverse relationship exists between prepregnancy BMI and success rates for vaginal birth after cesarean delivery. Pregnant women with class III obesity undergoing a trial of labor after previous cesarean delivery had greater rates of composite morbidity (prolonged hospital stay, endometritis, rupture, or dehiscence) and neonatal injury (fractures, brachial plexus injuries, and lacerations) compared with women with class III obesity who had elective repeat cesarean delivery, but the absolute frequency of morbidities was low.[20] Compared with normal-weight pregnant women, pregnant women with obesity have a significantly increased risk of postpartum atonic hemorrhage (bleeding greater than 1000 mL) after a vaginal delivery but not after cesarean delivery. Obesity is also a well-known risk factor for thromboembolism, with a linear effect as to the degree of obesity.[21]

The risk of surgical site infection after cesarean delivery can approach 20%. The risk of surgical site infection after cesarean delivery is highest among obese women. Compared with normal-weight women, there is an increased risk of surgical site infections.[22]

CONCLUSION

Although the management of obesity requires long-term approaches from societal, economic, and public health entities, as well as individual nutritional, medical, and behavioral modifications, these are not the focus of this chapter and this book. This chapter gives an overview of the effect of the obesity epidemic on the management outcomes of pregnant patients and emphasizes the increasing magnitude of the problem faced by providers in safety-net hospitals. Obesity increases the likelihood that a pregnant patient will require a cesarean delivery and then compounds the problem by increasing the likelihood of complications during and after the performance of that surgical intervention.

Compounding the difficulty of taking care of these patients is a cultural bias against overweight and obese women which is displayed in all aspects of mass media in the United States. It is not uncommon to hear medical personnel refer to these patients in a derogatory manner. Not infrequently providers of all stripes are reluctant to provide care. Facing this reality, the American College of Obstetricians and Gynecologists, in a recent committee opinion, published the following statement[23]:

"If physicians place value judgments on obesity and see this condition as different from other chronic health conditions or determinants, they are at risk of treating their obese patients with bias. If, however, obesity is seen as a modifiable risk factor, in the mold of hypertension, hypercholesterolemia, or smoking, physicians will be better able to objectively counsel and care for their obese patients in an ethical and effective manner."

REFERENCES

1. Purnell J. Epidemiology of obesity. 2018. Available at https://www.ncbi.nlm.nih.gov/books/NBK279167/. Accessed February 20, 2019.
2. Committee on Gynecologic Practice. Committee opinion no. 619: gynecologic surgery in the obese woman. *Obstet Gynecol*. 2015;125:274-278.
3. Sturm R. Increases in clinically severe obesity in the United States. 1986-2000. *Arch Intern Med*. 2003;103:219-224.
4. Jensen MD, Ryan DH, Apovian CM, et al. 2013 AHA/ACA/TOS guideline for the management of overweight and obesity in adults: a report of the American College of Cardiology/American Heart Association Task Force on Practice Guidelines and The Obesity Society. *J Am Coll Cardiol*. 2013. doi:10.106/j.jacc2013.11.004.
5. Afshin A, Forouzanfar MH, Reitsma MB, et al. Health effects of overweight and obesity in 195 countries over 25 years. *N Eng J Med*. 2017;377(1):13-27.
6. O'Brien KS, Latner JD, Ebneter D, Hunter JA. Obesity discrimination: the role of physical appearance, personal ideology, and anti-fat prejudice. *Int J Obes*. 2013;37:455-460.
7. Atlas S. Single Payer's Misleading Statistics. *Wall Str J*. December 18, 2018;A19.
8. Global BMI. Mortality Collaborative: body-mass index and all-cause mortality, individual-participant-data meta- analysis of 239 prospective studies in four continents. *Lancet*. 2016;388(10046):776-786.
9. National Obesity Rates and Trends. Available at https://stateofobesity.org/obesity-rates-trends-overview/.
10. WHO Expert Consultation. Appropriate body-mass index for Asian populations and its implications for policy intervention strategies. *Lancet*. 2004;363:157-163.
11. NHLBI Obesity Education Initiative Expert Panel on the Identification, Evaluation, and Treatment of Obesity in Adults (US). *Clinical Guidelines on the Identification, Evaluation, and Treatment of Overweight and Obesity in Adults*. Bethesda, MD: National Heart, Lung, and Blood Institute; 1998. Available at https://www.ncbi.nlm.nih.gov/books/NBK2003/.

12. Office of the Surgeon General (US), Office of Disease Prevention and Health Promotion (US), Centers for Disease Control and Prevention (US), National Institutes of Health (US). *The Surgeon General Call to Action to Prevent and Decrease Overweight and Obesity.* Rockville, MD: Office of the Surgeon General (US); 2001. Available at https://www.ncbi.nlm.nih.gov/books/NBK44206/.

13. Hales CH, Caroll MD, Fryar CD, Ogden CL. *Prevalence of obesity among adults and youths United States 2015 – 2016.* NCHS Data Report No. 288; 2017. Available at https://www.cdc.gov/nchs/data/databriefs/db288.pdf.

14. New Report Shows US Obesity Epidemic Continues to Worsen. American Academy of Family Physicians. October 15, 2018. Available at https://www.aafp.org/news/health-of-the-public/20181015obesityrpt.html.

15. NCD Risk Factor Collaboration. Worldwide trends in body-mass index, underweight, overweight, and obesity from 1975 to 2016: a pooled analysis of 2416 population-based measurement studies in 128.9 million children, adolescents, and adults. *Lancet.* December 2017;390:2627-2642.

16. Weiss JL, Malone FD, Emig D, et al. Obesity, obstetric complications and cesarean delivery rate- a population-based screening study. FASTER Research Consortium. *Am J Obstet Gynecol.* 2004;190:1091-1097.

17. Hull HR, Dinger MK, Knehans AW, Thompson DM, Fields DA. Impact of maternal body mass index on neonate birthweight and body composition. *Am J Obstet Gynecol.* 2008;198:416.

18. Cedergren MI. Maternal morbid obesity and the risk of adverse pregnancy outcome. *Obstet Gynecol.* 2004;103:219-224.

19. Norman SM, Tuuli MG, Odibo AO, Caughey AB, Roehi KA, Cahill AG. The effect of obesity on the first stage of labor. *Obstet Gynecol.* 2012;120:130-135.

20. Hibbard JU, Gilbert S, Landon MB, et al. Trial of labor or repeat cesarean delivery in women with morbid obesity and previous cesarean delivery. *Obstet Gynecol.* 2006;108:125-133.

21. Chu SY, Kim SY, Schmid CH, et al. Maternal obesity and risk of cesarean delivery: a meta-analysis. *Obes Rev.* 2007;8:385-394.

22. Bell J, Bell S, Vahratian A, Awonuga AO. Abdominal surgical incisions and perioperative morbidity among morbidly obese women undergoing cesarean delivery. *Eur J Obstet Gynecol Reprod Biol.* 2011;154:16-19.

23. Ethical Issues in the Care of the Obese Woman ACOG Committee Opinion 763. *Obstet Gynecol.* 2019;133:e90-e95.

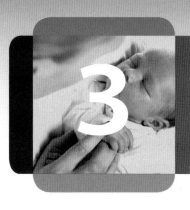

3

Normal Physiology of Placentation

Erin H. Burnett

INTRODUCTION

The placenta is a unique organ that has numerous functions; however, in order for the placenta to function appropriately, a gamut of precise processes need to occur. The development of the placenta begins at implantation and should be complete by the end of the first trimester.[1] The placenta's primary purpose involves exchange of oxygen and nutrients and the removal of waste. A properly attached placenta and therefore properly functioning placenta is vital, as it must deal with the large majority of uterine blood flow.

Overall, the placenta is a mysterious yet magnificent organ, and although we continue to learn more about it, there are still so many aspects that are puzzling and not fully explained. The aim of this chapter is to describe the "normal" aspect of implantation and placental development to help readers in understanding and recognizing abnormal placentation discussed in other chapters.

PREIMPLANTATION (FIGURE 3-1)

The fallopian tubes most frequently serve as the site of fertilization. The fertilized ovum (zygote) transitions to a solid mass of cells (morula) as it moves through the fallopian tube on its way to the uterus. The embryo has a protective covering called the zona pellucida, which serves as a protective coating during the transit. This coating prevents the embryo from sticking to the sides of the tube. Even before the embryo makes its way to the uterus, decidualization has already begun in the midsecretory phase of the menstrual cycle.[2] Rising progesterone levels halt proliferation and cause endometrial and stromal cells to begin to differentiate.[2] The glandular cells also prepare for implantation by producing secretory products and cytokines.[3,4] Stromal cells also play a role in preparation, and natural killer cells accumulate. The uterine vasculature is directed to have increased permeability, and the capillary network matures in preparation of implantation.[5] The overall process of decidualization provides maternal immune tolerance, along with protection to the fetus and regulation of placentation.[6]

The morula usually arrives in the uterus around 3 days post fertilization.[7] The morula becomes more organized at day 5 to 6 and is then referred to as a blastocyst, which contains an inner and outer cell mass. The outer cell mass, the *trophoblast*, forms the placenta and fetal membrane, and an inner cell mass, forms the embryo (Figure 3-2).[8]

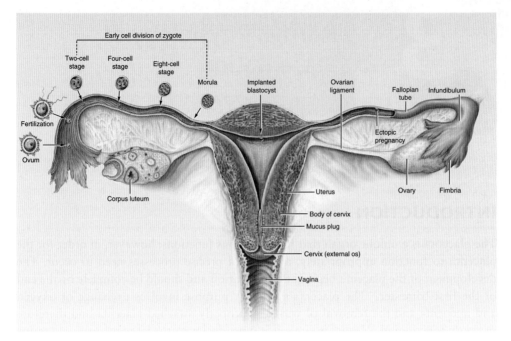

FIGURE 3-1 Normal female anatomy depicting the normal location for various stages of fertilization and implantation. (Reprinted with permission from the Anatomical Chart Company. "Infertility Anatomical Chart." Lippincott Williams & Wilkins; 2004.)

The blastocyst also has the very distinctive feature of a fluid filled cavity. This fluid helps the blastocyst expand and contract which allows it to "hatch" from the zona pellucida, therefore preparing it for implantation. After hatching, uterine secretions help support the embryo by providing oxygen and nutrients.[8] Due to the rapidly increasing demand of the embryo, these secretions will become inadequate within 24 hours; therefore, the cell must implant to survive.

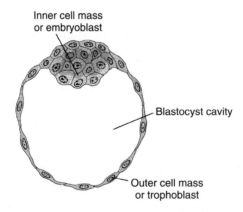

FIGURE 3-2 Blastocyst with outer trophoblast (green) and inner cell mass (blue) The inner cell mass gives rise to the entire embryo and is displaced to one pole of the blastocyst, the embryonic pole; the outer cell mass forms the outer layer of the blastocyst and contributes to development of the placenta. (Adapted from Sadler TW. *Langman's Essential Medical Embryology.* Wolters Kluwer Health and Pharma; 2004 [Figure 2-1].)

ANATOMY OF THE ENDOMETRIUM

While the blastocyst prepares to implant, estrogen and progesterone prepare the endometrium of the uterus. Stromal cells enlarge and become surrounded by edematous fluid and glycogen fills the glandular cells.[1] The *endometrium*, also known as the *decidua*, is made up of three layers and will be shed at the end of the pregnancy, the stratum compactum, stratum spongiosum, and stratus basalis. The surface layer (stratum compactum) has very few glands, but the middle, stratum spongiosum, contains many glands and vessels, which serve as the target for the invading blastocyst (Figure 3-3).[1]

STAGES OF IMPLANTATION

Successful implantation and invasion requires complex interaction between a receptive uterus and a mature and appropriately functioning blastocyst.[7] Attraction to certain regions of the endometrium occurs in response to molecular signals expressed on the respective surfaces. Implantation starts around day 6 to 7 and is thought to occur in three stages discussed below.

Stage 1: Apposition

The initial stage involves the initial contact with the endometrium. The blastocyst then rolls against the wall and adhesion of the blastocyst to the uterine wall occurs; this is referred to as *apposition*.[7] The trophoblast, outside layer of the blastocyst, proliferates and divides into layers, the cytotrophoblast and the syncytiotrophoblast. The inner layer, cytotrophoblast, forms the foundation of the chorionic villi and placenta. The outer layer, syncytiotrophoblast, secretes enzymes assisting with implantation and will expand into the placenta parenchyma (Figure 3-4).[8]

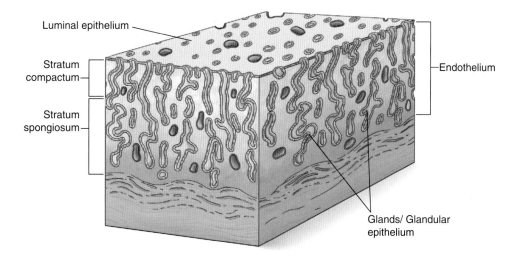

FIGURE 3-3 Endometrium layers of the uterus.

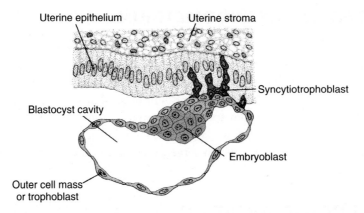

FIGURE 3-4 Blastocyst beginning implantation into the uterus. (Modified from Sadler TW. *Langman's Essential Medical Embryology.* © Wolters Kluwer Health and Pharma; 2004 [Figure 2-1].)

Stage 2: Adhesion

This second stage is known as "adhesion."[7] At day 7 to 8, the cells on the outside of the blastocyst show increased physical attraction and the trophectoderm, a trophoblast that has completed gastrulation, sticks to the uterine epithelium.

Stage 3: Invasion and Uteroplacental Circulation

The third stage known as "invasion" begins during day 8 to 9 and is characterized by the syncytiotrophoblasts penetrating the uterine epithelium (see Figure 3-5). The syncytiotrophoblasts provide the barrier to maternal blood and help regular oxygen and protein transport.[9] Invasion stage peaks between weeks 9 to 12 of pregnancy.

At day 10, the blastocyst should be completely buried in the subepithelium and the uterine epithelium has covered the implantation site.[10] Interstitial and

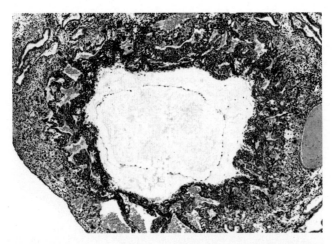

FIGURE 3-5 Implantation site at approximately 2 weeks of gestation. The finger-like trophoblastic projections represent primary stem villi and are closely associated with lacunae filled with maternal blood. Note that the endometrial surface has been reepithelialized by this stage of development (lower left).

endovascular invasion occur next as the cytotrophoblasts exude out of the tropho-blastic shell and then invade the endometrium and eventually the maternal uterine vasculature.[11]

This anchoring officially begins the process of placentation, by creating a utero-placental circulation through placing fetal trophoblasts directly in contact with mater-nal blood. Trophoblasts are thought to normally invade through the endometrium in the inner third of the myometrium.[12] The interstitial trophoblasts target the myome-trial tissue, and the endovascular trophoblast aim for remodeling the maternal spiral arteries.

Role of Regulatory Proteins and Decidual Natural Killer Cells in Successful Placentation

In order to assist in the process, proteases breakdown the basement membrane to allow stable anchoring.[13] Hepatocyte growth factor[14] and epidermal growth factor (EGF)[15] serve to stimulate trophoblast migration, while interferon-γ (IFN-γ) and transforming growth factor-β (TGFB) limit trophoblastic invasion.[16] Decidual nat-ural killer cells (dNKs) account for 70% of the immune cells recruited during this process, and they assist in regulating cellular interactions.[17] dNKs are thought to have significant contribution to successful placentation (see Figure 3-6). One main role includes expressing cytokines and chemokines, which signal to trophoblasts, therefore helping to regulate invasion.[18] dNKs also can influence uterine vascular cells via their expression of pro- and antiangiogenic factors.[18,19] In order for placentation and remodeling to be successful, a careful balance must be achieved between all the regulatory proteins.[14]

In addition, there are several additional cytokines, growth factors, steroid hor-mones, and immunological agents involved in this process of placentation.[13]

Uteroplacental Circulation

By day 13, the trophoblast erodes deep into the decidua forming vacuoles leading to lacunae. A low-resistance vascular network forms from the anastomoses between

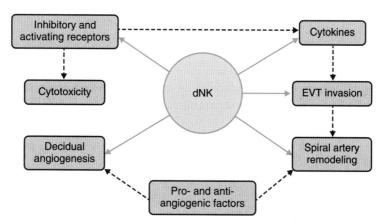

FIGURE 3-6 Possible roles of decidual natural killer cells (dNKs) in placentation and spiral artery remodeling. Direct effects are indicated by solid arrows, and indirect effects are indicated by dashed arrows.

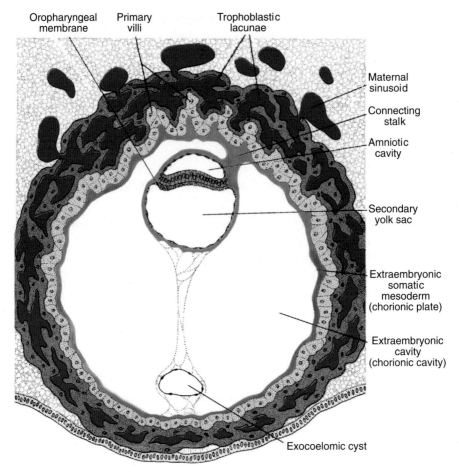

FIGURE 3-7 Diagram of 13-day blastocyst that erodes into the decidua forming vacuoles which lead to trophoblastic lacunae and uteroplacental circulation has begun. (Reprinted with permission from Sadler TW. *Langman's Medical Embryology*. 13th ed. © Wolters Kluwer Health and Pharma; 2014 [Figure 4-6].)

dilated spiral arteries and endometrial veins. This leads to the intervillous space which develops out of the lacunar spaces and therefore establishes uteroplacental circulation.[8] Formation of primary villi with their close association with the maternal vasculature can also be seen in Figure 3-7.

In the process of the chorionic villi implanting into the spongiosus layer of the uterine decidua, there is a natural plane of separation.[12] This plane lies superior to the decidua basalis and allows prompt separation of the placenta after delivery.

CLINICAL PEARL

The decidua itself provides a barrier to pathological myometrial invasion.[13] A *deficiency of decidualized* tissue is thought to contribute to abnormal placentation.[20]

A summary of the implantation process is depicted in Figure 3-8.

SECOND AND THIRD WEEK OF PLACENTAL DEVELOPMENT

Villous development continues (Figure 3-9), as primary mesenchymal villi become secondary villi.[8] While the placenta is beginning to form, the inner cell mass becomes a bilaminar disk containing an epiblast and a hypoblast. The epiblast will differentiate via gastrulation into three primitive germ layers: ectoderm, endoderm, and mesoderm, and to the extraembryonic mesoderm of the visceral yolk sac, the allantois, and the amnion. This mesoderm differentiates into blood vessels by day 21 after fertilization.[8] Those vessels form the connection to the embryo via the umbilical cord; this is considered tertiary villi. Villi are anchored to maternal decidua while others float in the lacuna, but the maternal and fetal circulations always stay separated via the layer of trophoblasts.

Continuation of Vascular Development

First trimester placentas are dominated by *villous cytotrophoblasts*. Over time, cells are turned over to the *syncytiotrophoblast*, and therefore, later gestation has few cytotrophoblasts as it is dominated by syncytiotrophoblasts.[8] Increases in the length and size of the villi leads to the placentas increasing in thickness through the end of the fourth month of gestation.[1] Thickness typically remains stable at that time; however, placenta circumference will continue to increase throughout the remainder of the pregnancy. Looking for a thin cytotrophoblast layer on electron microscope would help confirm a placenta >5 months.[1] At term, syncytiotrophoblasts have a surface area of 12 to 14 m^2 by term.[8] In areas of high altitude, the surface area is increased leading to overall larger placentas.

EARLY PLACENTA FORMATION: IMPORTANCE OF VESSEL REMODELING

In the first few weeks of pregnancy, spiral artery remodeling takes place in order to accommodate a developing fetus. This process involves changing the arteries from low-flow, high resistance to high-flow, low resistance.[21] The process of these changes occurs in precise stages and ultimately remodels the vessel walls, increasing the vessel diameter and allowing increased blood flow (Figure 3-10). Although the full mechanism of these actions has not been completely discovered, a number of individual maternal and fetal processes have been discovered which contribute to these crucial steps (Figure 3-11 algorithm).[9] Cells involved include but are not limited to IFN-ɣ, macrophages, and pro- and antiangiogenic factors.[9] After spiral artery remodeling has completed, the dNKs disperse leading to their numbers at term being low.[22] Knowledge of these complex processes continues to increase and makes it more evident of the multiple stages that can be compromised during placentation and remodeling. Figure 3-12A and B depicts pathology specimens of normal cellular invasion; these can be contrasted with abnormal invasion discussed in Chapter 4.

Overall, the invasion process peaks between weeks 9 through 12 and is thought to be a vital role in normal placentation.[12]

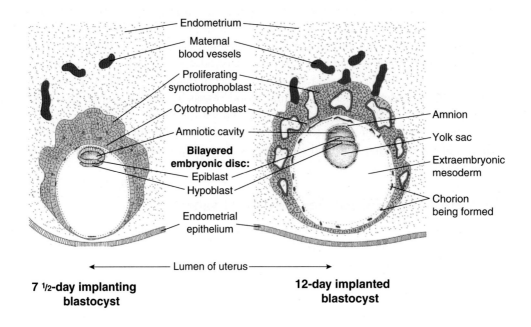

**7 ½-day implanting
blastocyst**

**12-day implanted
blastocyst**

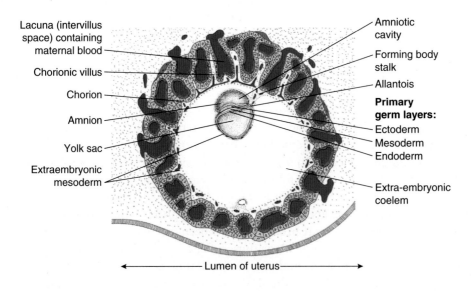

16-day embryo

FIGURE 3-8 Human placental development. Blastocyst implants inside the endometrium of the
uterus.

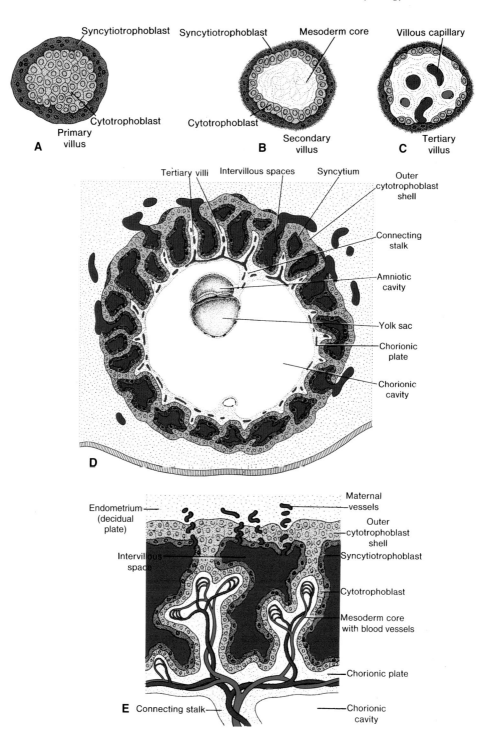

FIGURE 3-9 Stages of vessel formation from primary villus to an extensive network of blood vessels allowing oxygen exchange. (From Sadler TW. *Langman's Medical Embryology.* 13th ed. Wolters Kluwer Health and Pharma; 2014.)

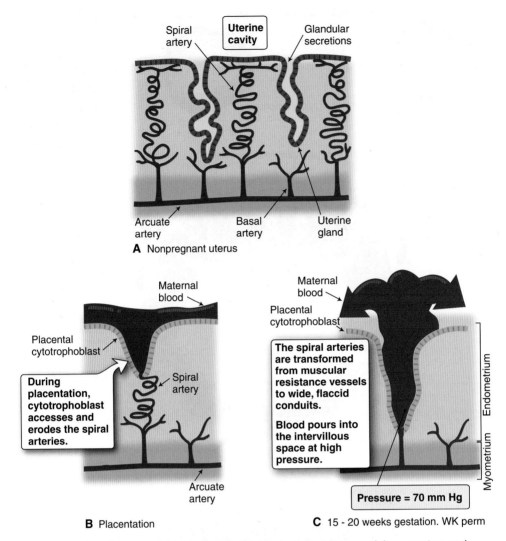

FIGURE 3-10 Cellular interactions involved in decidual spiral artery remodeling, erosion, and invasion of spiral arteries during placentation. (Modified from Preston RR, Wilson T. *Lippincott Illustrated Reviews: Physiology.* Lippincott, Williams & Wilkins/Wolters Kluwer; 2012.)

PLACENTAL DEVELOPMENT AND CHARACTERISTICS IN SECOND AND THIRD TRIMESTER

The overall vessel development over the gestation proceeds with vasculogenesis followed by branching.[8] When looking at the maternal surface, the placenta is divided into sections called *cotyledons*, and each is supplied by a major branch of the umbilical artery (Figure 3-13). The grooves on the maternal side prevent excessive lateral flow within the intervillous space and help anchor the placenta.[1] The fetal surface of the placenta is flat and smooth with the umbilical cord, in most cases, entering near the center and at a 90° angle (Figure 3-14). These vessels in the umbilical cord enter the placenta and divide into secondary vessels and then to tertiary vessels.[8] These disseminate into the main-stem *villi*, to the intermediate villi and finally to the terminal villi which serves as the

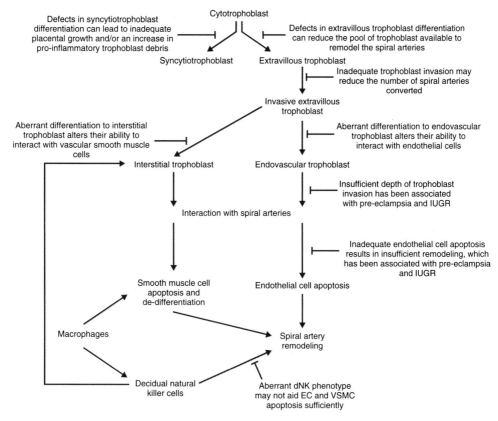

Cytotrophoblast

Defects in syncytiotrophoblast differentiation can lead to inadequate placental growth and/or an increase in pro-inflammatory trophoblast debris

Defects in extravillous trophoblast differentiation can reduce the pool of trophoblast available to remodel the spiral arteries

Syncytiotrophoblast   Extravillous trophoblast

Inadequate trophoblast invasion may reduce the number of spiral arteries converted

Invasive extravillous trophoblast

Aberrant differentiation to interstitial trophoblast alters their ability to interact with vascular smooth muscle cells

Aberrant differentiation to endovascular trophoblast alters their ability to interact with endothelial cells

Interstitial trophoblast   Endovascular trophoblast

Insufficient depth of trophoblast invasion has been associated with pre-eclampsia and IUGR

Interaction with spiral arteries

Inadequate endothelial cell apoptosis results in insufficient remodeling, which has been associated with pre-eclampsia and IUGR

Smooth muscle cell apoptosis and de-differentiation   Endothelial cell apoptosis

Macrophages

Spiral artery remodeling

Decidual natural killer cells

Aberrant dNK phenotype may not aid EC and VSMC apoptosis sufficiently

FIGURE 3-11 Algorithm of the stages of trophoblastic differentiation and invasion. dNK, decidual natural killer cell; EC, endothelial cell; IUGR, intrauterine growth restriction; VSMC, vascular smooth muscle cell. (From Cartwright JE, Fraser R, Leslie K, et al. Remodeling at the maternal-fetal interface: relevance to human pregnancy disorders. *Reproduction.* 2010;140:803-813.)

exchange unit. Each terminal villi contains three to five capillaries all of which consists of loops and sinusoids. This increased surface area reduces resistance, therefore enhancing exchange. Villi grow and develop until term; however, as the gestation approaches term, some villi begin to degenerate and fibrin-like material collects between the villi.[1]

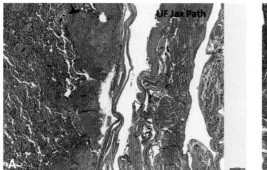
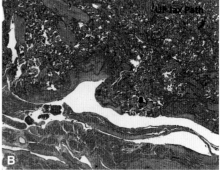

FIGURE 3-12 Images depict pathology slide of normal placentation at the cellular level. Normal villi implant within the decidua and a clear border is seen between the villi and the myometrium. (Slides Courtesy of Pathology Department, University of Florida.)

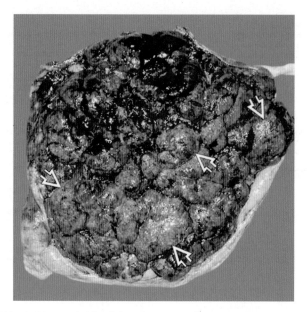

FIGURE 3-13 Maternal side of the placenta with arrows showing cotyledons.

The villi of the placenta have direct contact with the maternal blood and are composed of a single layer of *trophoblasts* that serve as the barrier between the maternal blood and fetal vessels.[23] Maternal blood flows through the spiral arteries and into the intervillous space where it baths the *syncytiotrophoblasts* (Figure 3-15). Fetal blood then enters the arteries of the basal surface of the placenta. These arteries branch into capillaries, and then after gaining oxygen and nutrients, the blood exits the placenta via the umbilical vein.[23]

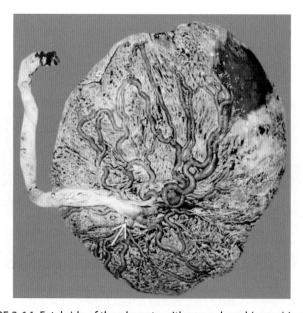

FIGURE 3-14 Fetal side of the placenta with normal cord (arrow) insertion.

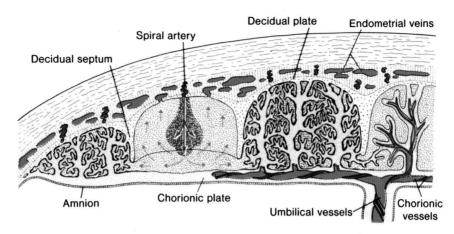

FIGURE 3-15 Sagittal diagram depicting the inner workings of a normal placenta.

FUNCTIONS OF A NORMAL PLACENTA

Numerous processes must occur for the placenta to function properly. The three main functions of the placenta include

- exchange of nutrients and waste between mother and fetus,
- production and excretion of hormones, and
- sustainment of an immunological barrier.[1]

The placenta serves as the lifeline for the fetus by providing all the oxygen and nutrients, in addition to filtering out harmful toxins. These processes are vital to helping the fetus grow appropriately and decreasing harm to the unborn child.

PLACENTAL SEPARATION AND DELIVERY

After infants are born, the placenta(s) must be delivered as well, known as the third stage of labor. In the presence of normal placentation, contractions of the myometrium after delivery cause a shearing action between the surface of the placenta and uterus, and the placenta typically separates easily. This process is usually completed within 30 minutes of infant delivery. This contraction of the myometrium also constricts the vascular supply and decreases hemorrhage risk.[12]

CLINICAL PEARL

Once the placenta has delivered, it is important for the delivering provider to examine the placenta to ensure all the cotyledons are present.

Anatomy and Inspection of the Delivered Placenta

Gross description of a normal full-term placenta includes a round, disk-shaped, or oval structure measuring 18 × 20 cm in diameter and approximately 2 cm thick.[24] Typical weight ranges from 400 to 600 g, and there exists a wide variety of sizes and shapes. This gamut can partly be explained by different races, altitude, maternal disease, social habits, ie, tobacco and drug use, and variations starting at implantation. The cord is normally inserted near the center of the disk.

Theories of Abnormal Placenta Insertion

In 7% of cases, a marginal placenta insertion (within 2 cm of the placental edge) is detected, and 1% of the time, the cord inserts into the membranes, known as velamentous.[25] There are two competing theories on what leads the cord to not implant in the center. One thought suggests that at the time of implantation, the embryo had a less than perfect central position; therefore, when the location of the cord was established, it is more lateral. If the location of the cord gets established on the surface of the endometrium, this will lead to the cord inserting on the membranes. An alternative hypothesis suggests that the forming placenta recognizes that area of initial implantation was less than optimal for development. Therefore, much like a placenta previa usually moves to areas of better blood flow via trophotropism and grows more in one direction, the expansion of the newly implanted placenta may occur to one side rather than in a uniform centrifugal manner, leading to a marginal or velamentous cord insertion.

Further Inspection of Fetal Side and Maternal Side

Upon further inspection of the placenta, the membranes attach to the edge of the placental disk, and the amnion and chorion are slightly adherent and therefore can be separated with tissue forceps. When examining the placenta itself, there is a fetal side and a maternal side, as discussed above and noted in Figures 3-13 and 3-14. The fetal side is noted to be blue due to the fetal villous blood content, as uterine contractions expelled most of the maternal blood. The maternal surface consists of multiple cotyledons, with partial or complete septa between them. Decidual cells and cellular trophoblasts make up these septa. The decidua basalis has a grayish color to it and is in close communication with fibrin which contains calcifications, characterizing its level of maturity.

SUGGESTED VIDEOS

What is the placenta?—Definition, Development and Function (full video not available). https://study.com/academy/lesson/what-is-the-placenta-definition-development-function.html

The Placenta: Its Development and Function. https://www.youtube.com/watch?v=bped-RVWsLk

REFERENCES

1. Ahokas R, McKinney E. Development and physiology of the placenta and membranes. *Glob Libr Womens Med.* 2008. doi:10.3842/GLOWM.10101. http://www.glowm.com/section_view/heading/development+and+physiology+of+the+placenta+and+membranes/item/101.
2. Dockery P, Li TC, Rogers AW, et al. The ultrastructure of the glandular epithelium in the timed endometrial biopsy. *Hum Reprod.* 1988;3:826-834.
3. Cullinan EB, Abbondanzo SJ, Anderson PS, et al. Leukemia inhibitory factor (LIF) and LIF receptor expression in human endometrium suggests a potential autocrine/paracrine function in regulating embryo implantation. *Proc Natl Acad Sci.* 1996;93:3115-3120. doi:10.1073/pnas.93.7.3115.

4. Tabibzadeh S, Kong QF, Babaknia A, et al. Progressive rise in the expression of interleukin-6 in human endometrium during menstrual cycle is initiated during implantation window. *Hum Reprod.* 1995;10:2793-2799.

5. Demir R, Yaba A, Huppertz B. Vasculogenesis and angiogenesis in the endometrium during menstrual cycle and implantation. *Acta Histochem.* 2010;112:203-214. doi:10.1016/j.placenta.2009.12.027.

6. Salker M, Teklenburg G, Molokhia M, et al. Natural selection of human embryos: impaired decidualization of endometrium disables embryo-maternal interactions and causes recurrent pregnancy loss. *PLoS One.* 2010;5:e10287. doi:10.1371/journal.pone.0010287.

7. Norwitz ER. Defective implantation and placentation: laying the blueprint for pregnancy complications. *Reproductive Biomed Online.* 2006;13(4):591-599.

8. Roberts V, Myatt L. Placental development and physiology. *Up-to-date.* Available at https://discovery.lifemapsc.com/library/review-of-medical-embryology/chapter-41-placental-physiology. Accessed June 2018.

9. Cartwright JE, Fraser R, Leslie K, et al. Remodeling at the maternal-fetal interface: relevance to human pregnancy disorders. *Reproduction.* 2010;140:803-813.

10. Benirschke K, Kaufmann P. *Early Development of the Human Placenta. Pathology of the Human Placenta.* NY: Springer-Verlag; 1991:13-21.

11. Pijnenborg R, Robertson WB, Brosens I, et al. Review article: trophoblast invasion and the establishment of haemochorial placentation in man and laboratory animals. *Placenta.* 1981;2:71-91.

12. Bauer ST, Bonanno C. Abnormal placentation. *Semin Perinatol.* 2009;33(2):88-95.

13. Cramer SF, Heller DS. Placenta accrete and placenta increta: an approach to pathogenesis based on trophoblastic differentiation pathway. *Pediatr Dev Pathol.* 2016;19:320-333.

14. Cartwright JE, Tse WK, Whitley GS. Hepatocyte growth factor induced human trophoblast motility involves phosphatidylinositol-3-kinase, mitogen-activated protein kinase, and inducible nitric oxide synthase. *Exp Cell Res.* 2002;279:219-226.

15. Staun-Ram E, Goldman S, Shaley E. p53 Mediates epidermal growth factor (EGF) induction of MMP-2 transcription and trophoblast invasion. *Placenta.* 2009;30:1029-1036.

16. Knofler M. Critical growth factors and signaling pathways controlling human trophoblastic invasion. *Int J Dev Biol.* 2010;54:269-280.

17. Moffett-King A. Natural killer cells and pregnancy. *Nat Rev Immunol.* 2002;2:656-663.

18. Hanna I, Goldman-Wohl D, Hamani Y, et al. Decidual NK cells regulate key developmental processes at the human fetal-maternal interface. *Nat Med.* 2006;12:1065-1074.

19. Lash GE, Schiessl B, Kirkley M, et al. Expression of angiogenic growth factors by uterine natural killer cells during early pregnancy. *J Leukoc Biol.* 2006;80:572-580.

20. Khong TY. The pathology of placenta accrete, a worldwide epidemic. *J Clin Pathol.* 2008:611243-611246.

21. Brosens IA, Robertson WB, Dixon HG. The role of spiral arteries in the pathogenesis of preeclampsia. *Obstet Gynecol Annu.* 1972;1:177-191.

22. Williams PJ, Searle RF, Robsen SC. Decidual leucocyte populations in early to late gestation normal human pregnancy. *J Reprod Immunol.* 2009;82:24-31.

23. McNanley T, Woods J. Placental physiology. *J Glob Libr Women's Med.* 2008. doi:10.3843/GLOWM.10195. http://www.glowm.com/section_view/heading/placental%20physiology/item/195.

24. Benirschke K. *Normal early development.* In: *Creasy & Resnik Maternal Fetal Based Principles.* 7th ed. Philadelphia, PA: Elsevier Saunders; 2014:37-46.

25. Woodward PJ, Kennedy A, Sohaey R, et al. *Diagnostic Imaging Obstetrics.* 3rd ed. Philadelphia: Elsevier; 2016:814-815.

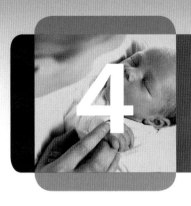

4 Abnormal Placentation after Cesarean Delivery

Erin H. Burnett

INTRODUCTION AND STATISTICS

Cesareans continue to be the most commonly performed procedure in the United States accounting for about 32% of the births nationwide. These critical issues of abnormal placentation will likely become more prevalent. Thankfully ultrasound technology has vastly improved making diagnoses easier, but facilities must still continue to train ultrasound teams to carefully watch for these abnormal placentations, especially in the setting of previous cesareans or other uterine surgeries. This chapter will discuss the various types of abnormal placentation including low-lying placenta, placenta previa, placenta accreta spectrum (PAS) which refers to the creta spectrum (accreta, increta, and percreta), and cesarean scar pregnancy (CSP).

In 2015 and 2016, nearly 4 million births per year were registered in the United States.[1] This number has declined slightly since the most recent peak in 2007 when over 4.3 million births were registered. The cesarean delivery rate has been relatively stable around 32% for the past 8 years.[1] Before 2009, the cesarean delivery rate had steadily increased every year since 1996 when it was 20.7%.[1] The "low-risk" cesarean rate has been steady at 25% to 27% in the past 7 years.[1] "Low risk" implies a single-ton, term (37 weeks gestation or beyond), and cephalic presentation having a cesarean for their first pregnancy.[1] The VBAC (vaginal birth after cesarean) rate in 2016 was only 12.4% (Table 4-1).[1]

RISK FACTORS ASSOCIATED WITH CESAREAN MORBIDITY

As cesareans rates rise over the years, so too has the morbidity associated with them. The majority of uterine scars heal normally; however, some can be found to have an anterior uterine wall deficiency.[2] Increasing number of prior cesarean increases the surface area of the scar and the risk of fibrosis, which has known poor vascular-ity, and hence raises the risk of inappropriate healing.[2,3] Hence, the uterine scar left behind after a cesarean increases the risk of PAS, scar dehiscence, and a rare form of ectopic pregnancy know as a cesarean scar pregnancy (CSP).[4] Studies estimate that of the cases where the placenta implants on the cesarean scar, 30% to 40% have abnormal placentation.[5,6] This exponentially increases the risk for hemorrhage and hysterectomy.

TABLE 4-1 Births by Method of Delivery and Race and Hispanic Origin of Mother in the United States (2010-2016)

Year and Race and Hispanic Origin	Number							Percent			
	All Births Total	Vaginal Total^a	Vaginal After Previous Cesarean	Cesarean Total^b	Cesarean Primary	Cesarean Low-risk^c	Not Stated	Cesarean Total^d	Cesarean Primary^e	Cesarean Low-risk^f	Vaginal Birth After Previous Cesarean Delivery^g
All Races and Origins^h											
2016	3,945,875	2,684,803	75,244	1,258,581	728,500	329,614	2491	31.9	21.8	25.7	12.4
2015	3,978,497	2,703,504	—	1,272,503	—	331,982	2490	32.0	—	25.8	—
2014	3,988,076	2,699,951	—	1,284,551	—	337,086	3574	32.2	—	26.0	—
2013	3,932,181	2,642,892	—	1,284,339	—	344,405	4950	32.7	—	26.8	—
2012	3,952,841	2,650,744	—	1,296,070	—	355,942	6027	32.8	—	27.2	—
2011	3,953,590	2,651,428	—	1,293,267	—	359,669	8895	32.8	—	27.2	—
2010	3,999,386	2,680,947	—	1,309,182	—	368,523	9257	32.8	—	27.5	—
Non-hispanic, Single Race (2016)^i:											
White	2,056,332	1,419,788	37,442	635,588	379,240	172,006	956	30.9	21.5	24.7	12.8
Black	558,622	357,859	11,763	200,460	117,410	50,287	303	35.9	25.4	30.3	12.4
Hispanic^j	918,447	627,095	17,847	290,832	153,462	67,278	520	31.7	20.1	25.1	11.5

— Comparable data not available for the 50 states and District of Columbia for 2010 to 2015 because not all reporting areas had adopted the 2003 US Standard Certificate of Live Birth.

a Includes unknown type of vaginal delivery; see Technical Notes.

b Includes unknown type of cesarean delivery; see Technical Notes.

c Low-risk cesarean is defined as singleton, term (37 completed weeks or more of gestation based on the obstetric estimate), cephalic, cesarean deliveries to women having a first birth.

d Percentage of all live births delivered by cesarean.

e Primary cesarean rate is the number of births to women having a cesarean delivery per 100 births to women without a previous cesarean.

f Low-risk cesarean rate is the number of singleton, term (37 wk or more of gestation based on the obstetric estimate), cephalic, cesarean deliveries to women having a first birth per 100 women delivering singleton, term, cephalic, first births.

g Vaginal birth after cesarean delivery rate is the number of births to women having a vaginal delivery per 100 births to women with a previous cesarean delivery.

h Includes births to race and origin groups not shown separately, such as Hispanic single-race white, Hispanic single-race black, and non-Hispanic multiple-race women, as well as births with origin not stated.

i Race and Hispanic origin are reported separately on birth certificates; persons of Hispanic origin may be of any race. In this table, non-Hispanic women are classified by race. Race categories are consistent with 1997 Office of Management and Budget standards; see Technical Notes. Single race is defined as only one race reported on the birth certificate.

j Includes all persons of Hispanic origin of any race; see Technical Notes.

Reprinted with permission from Centers for Disease Control and Prevention. National Vital Statistics System, Natality. https://www.cdc.gov/nchs/nvss/index.htm.

Other uterine surgeries, besides cesareans, also contribute to the problem and include uterine curettage, hysteroscopy, myomectomy, endometrial ablation, and uterine artery embolization.[4,7] All of these surgeries cause damage to or a deficiency of decidualized tissue and an increase in fibrosis at the scar site, hence increasing the risk of abnormal placentation.[4,7] In addition, prior pelvic or whole body radiation or chemo therapy all have an increase incidence of accreta pointing to the theory of damaged decidua in these cases as well.[8-10] However, defective decidualized tissue cannot be the only cause as many pathology specimens are found to have normal decidualization.[11,12]

Multiple prior surgeries also compromise normal healing and lead to increased surface area of damaged tissue thus increasing the risk for abnormal placentation in subsequent pregnancies.[13-15] Just like any wound, repeated trauma leads to a disruption in the healing process. Cesarean scar healing can be compared to skin healing where the highly vascular granulation tissue is replaced by avascular scar tissue.[16] In patients with previous cesareans, the risk of abnormal placentation is fourfold higher if a central or anterior placenta previa is identified compared to a posterior previa.[17]

Downes identified a prelabor cesarean delivery, versus an intrapartum cesarean as a risk factor for previa, quoting a 2.62 odds ratio.[18] In addition, surgical techniques used for closure may affect one's risk. Closing the hysterotomy with a single layer versus a double layer results in a noninverting suture and may lead to deficient postoperative healing and therefore result in scar defects.[14]

IMPLANTATION SITES

Placenta location is typically determined for the first time during the anatomy scan around 18 to 20 weeks, unless a patient presents earlier for vaginal bleeding or other indications. The physical location of placental implantation should be described in one of three ways: previa, low-lying, and normal (usually anterior or posterior). In the past, during the preultrasound times, terms such as marginal, incomplete, and partial were used.[19] These terms are very ambiguous and subjective, hence consistent classification was lacking. In addition, the management did not change between these various "types."

TRANSVAGINAL ULTRASOUND AND IDENTIFICATION OF INTERNAL CERVICAL OS

Now that ultrasound is readily available, the location of the placenta can be determined by a transvaginal ultrasound (Figure 4-1A-D). After identifying the internal cervical os, the linear distance from the os to the edge of the placenta should be determined.[19]

- Previa: placenta covers the os to any degree
- Low-lying: the placenta does not cover the os, but lies within 2 cm of the os
- Normal: implies the placenta is greater than 2 cm away from the cervical os

Location should be determined at the time of the anatomy scan (18-24 weeks).[19] If there is concern via transabdominal ultrasound for a previa or low-lying placenta, then a transvaginal ultrasound should be performed for confirmation. For those patients who have a low-lying placenta or a placenta previa, the most common management is to reimage the location in the mid-third trimester. Some authors suggest that a low-lying

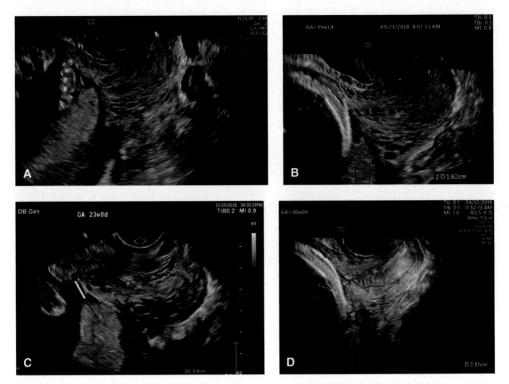

FIGURE 4-1 A-D, Depict various placenta locations. A, Placenta previa, B and C, low-lying placentas, D, normal location. Red/horizontal arrow shows the internal cervical os. Blue/vertical arrow points to edge of the placenta. The linear distance measured is reported (yellow line).

of at least 1 cm away does not need to be reimaged as the risk of complications is low.[19] Patients should be reassured that many abnormal placentations will resolve by the time of delivery.[19] The lower uterine segment grows and develops, and the overall blood supply in this area is not ideal for placental growth, therefore as the placenta grows with gestation, it is more apt to grow toward the fundus and away from the lower uterine segment as it seeks better blood supply.[19] Some believe that atrophy of the cells over the os occurs and therefore contributes to the resolution of previas (Table 4-2).[19]

MANAGEMENT DURING PREGNANCY

Women with placenta previa or vaginal bleeding in pregnancy should partake in pelvic rest; however, there is insufficient evidence to support bed rest.[19]

As previously discussed, most placentas initially implanted over or near the cervix will move with time and careful follow-up is generally acceptable. *However, patients experiencing signs of preterm labor and or vaginal bleeding should seek care immediately.*

Typical management of various placenta implantation sites can be seen in Figure 4-2.

Although the majority of patients with a low-lying placenta located 1 to 10 mm from the os result in cesareans, a patient should be counseled that vaginal deliveries are potentially still an option however there are increased risks (Table 4-3). These risks should be included in the counseling that occurs ideally before the onset of labor.

TABLE 4-2   Persistence of Placenta Previa according to Gestational Age at Ultrasound Detection

Type of Previa and prior cesarean	Gestational age at ultrasound detection (weeks)				
	15-19	20-23	24-27	28-31	32-35
Incomplete previa*, no prior cesarean	6	11	12	35	39
Incomplete previa*, prior cesarean	7	50	40	38	63
Complete previa, no prior cesarean	20	45	56	89	90
Complete previa, prior cesarean	41	73	84	88	89

*Note this study was prior to the reclassification of the placenta locations. Incomplete previa defined as inferior edge of the placenta partially covering the internal os.

Modified from Dashe JS, McIntire DD, Ramus RM, Santos-Ramos R, Twickler DM. Persistence of placenta previa according to gestational age at ultrasound detection. *Obstet Gynecol.* 2002;99:692-697; Becker RH, Vonk R, Mende BC, Ragosch V, Entezami M. The relevance of placental location at 20-23 gestational weeks for prediction of placenta previa at delivery: evaluation of 8650 cases. *Ultrasound Obstet Gynecol.* 2001;17:496-501; and Oppenheimer L, Holmes P, Simpson N, Dabrowski A. Diagnosis of low-lying placenta: can migration in the third trimester predict outcome? *Ultrasound Obstet Gynecol.* 2001;18:100-102.[20-22]

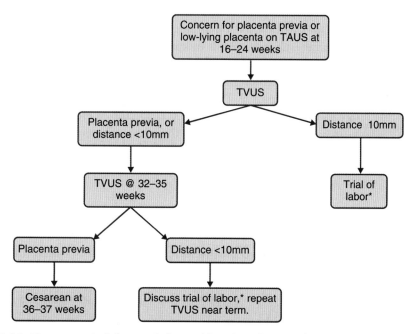

FIGURE 4-2 Management of abnormal placental locations. Distance: linear measurement from placental edge to internal cervical os. TAUS: transabdominal ultrasound, TVUS, transvaginal ultrasound. *Only after careful discussion with the patient and ensuring no contraindications. (Modified with permission from Son M, Grobman WA. Placental disorders. In: Berghella V, ed. *Obstetric Evidence Based Guidelines.* 3rd ed. New York: © CRC Press, Taylor & Francis Group; 2017:299-307. From original data in Spong CY, Mercer BM, D'alton M, et al. Timing of indicated late-preterm and early-term birth. *Obstet Gynecol.* 2011;118(2 Pt 1):323-333. doi:10.1097/AOG.0b013e3182255999.[23])

TABLE 4-3 Outcomes with Low-lying Placentas based on Distance between Cervical Os and Placenta Edge from Vergani results

Outcomes	Distance Between Internal Cervical Os and Placental Edge		
	1-10 mm	**11-20 mm**	**OR**
Cesarean	75%	31%	6.7
Antepartum hemorrhage	29%	3%	11.5
Postpartum hemorrhage	21%	10%	2.3
Blood loss at delivery	662 mL	510 mL	

Postpartum hemorrhage: defined as 500, 1000, respectively, for vaginal and cesarean study performed with old postpartum hemorrhage blood loss criteria OR: Odds ration.

Data from Vergani P, Ornaghi S, Pozzi I, et al. Placenta previa: distance to internal os and mode of delivery. *Am J Obstet Gynecol.* 2009;201:266.e1-266.e5.[24]

PLACENTA CRETA

The incidence of diagnosed placenta cretas has increased tenfold over the past 50 years, mostly due to the dramatic increase in cesarean rates over the past decades.[25] Current data indicate 1:300 to 2500 pregnancies have placenta creta.[26] The true incidence is complicated due to an underdiagnosis in pathology specimens and an overdiagnosis by clinical features, hence the true incidence is unknown.[25]

Abnormal placentation is a major cause of pregnancy complications and 50% to 65% of obstetrical hysterectomies occur due to postpartum hemorrhage in the setting of abnormal placentation.[27,28] The antepartum diagnosis can be challenging, and only histological evidence can confirm the suspicion.[19] However, absence of abnormal villous invasion does not exclude the creta spectrum from diagnosis; therefore, the diagnosis is often made clinically. The biggest risk factors for cretas include prior uterine surgery and the presence of a placenta previa (Table 4-4).[26]

TABLE 4-4 Risk of Accreta Based on Presence or Absence of Placenta Previa and the Number of Prior Cesareans

Cesarean Number	Placenta previa	No previa
First (primary)	3.3	0.03
Second	11	0.2
Third	40	0.1
Fourth	61	0.8
Fifth	67	0.8
Sixth or more	67	4.7

Modified with permission from Society for Maternal-Fetal Medicine. Quality of evidence: placenta accreta. *Am J Obstet Gynecol.* 2010;203:430-439.[29]

Accreta Spectrum Pathology

Abnormal placentation includes the creta spectrum: accreta, increta, and percreta, along with cesarean scar pregnancies. Current studies indicate the incidence of various degrees of invasive placentas within the creta spectrum[25,26]:

Accreta (75%-82%): attachment to the uterine myometrium but no invasion (Figure 4-3A and B)

Increta (12%-15%): invasion into the myometrium but not beyond the serosa (Figure 4-4A-C)

Percreta (5%-6%): invasion beyond the uterine serosa (Figure 4-5)

Pathogenesis of Cretas

The primary defect leading to abnormal placentation has yet to be elucidated however several theories of the pathogenesis exist. These include a primary defect in the decidua, abnormal remodeling within the maternal vasculature, excessive invasion of the trophoblast, or a combination of these.[30,31] Normal placentation as noted in the previous chapter[3] has decidualized endometrial stroma which allows placenta separation via shearing as the uterine myometrium contracts and therefore separates from the noncontracting placenta.[30] A prevailing hypothesis for placenta cretas speculate about an endometrial-myometrial interface defect leading to the failure of normal decidualization at the level of the uterine scar.[32] This defect allows trophoblasts to invade beyond the superficial myometrium resulting in villous development in the muscle layer. In placenta creta with the absence of the decidua, the normal plane of separation is lacking therefore causing adherent placenta and increasing the risk of postpartum hemorrhage and hence hysterectomy.[30] However, the decidual deficiency is not thought to fully explain the mechanism, and some authors hypothesize that this results from placental invasion and destruction.[12]

Excessive implantation may play a role as well. The normal implantation was previously described but involves trophoblasts invading the endometrium and the superficial myometrium in addition to spiral artery remodeling.[30] Smooth muscle within the arterial wall becomes replaced by trophoblasts which leads to a dilated lumina with hyalinized walls.[30]

In the creta spectrum, studies have noted defective and excessive invasion and remodeling.[12,33-35] Therefore, cretas appear to result from an improper interaction between the maternal tissues and the trophoblast in early placenta formation, coupled with the formation of abnormal uteroplacental circulation.[34,35] This leads to excessive invasion into the uterus and therefore adherent placenta.[34,35] Tantbirojn reviewed 49 cases and compared findings between creta and noncreta cases (Table 4-5).

Cases with creta were significantly more likely to have had uterine surgery and to have remodeled vessels. All cases of creta demonstrated an absence of decidua basilis, as the chorionic villi had direct contact with the myometrium.[30]

Tantbirojn also found that creta specimens displayed physiological change within the vessels and had notable vascular remodeling deeper into the myometrium, hence evidence of deeper trophoblastic invasion. Noncreta cases showed only a superficial layer of the myometrium with vessels, and they were completely remodeled.[30] Normally remodeled vessels consist of dilated lumens with walls that are completely

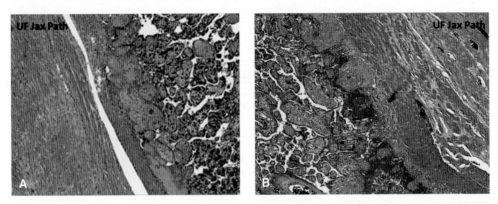

FIGURE 4-3 A and B, Accreta. Villi attach directly to the myometrium without invasion.

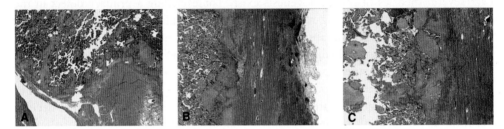

FIGURE 4-4 A-C, Increta. Villi invade deep into the myometrium.

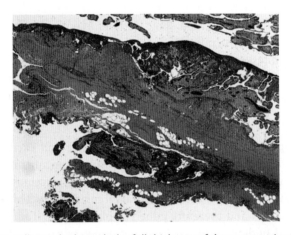

FIGURE 4-5 Percreta. Villi invade through the full thickness of the myometrium to the serosa (lower edge of image).

replaced by trophoblasts within a fibrinoid matrix.[30] This remodel serves to convert high-resistance, low-capacitance spiral arteries into vessels that are more conducive to the growing needs of a fetus, therefore low resistance and high capacitance.[30] In normally implanted placentas, these vessels remain confined to the inner one-third to one-half of the myometrium and are completed by the end of the first trimester. He

TABLE 4-5 Clinicopathological Characteristics in Cases of Creta Versus Noncreta[30]

Characteristics	Cases With Placenta Creta (*n* = 38)	Cases With No Placenta Creta (*n* = 11)	P Value
Age (mean ± S.D.) (range)	36.29 ± 5.54 (26-50)	33.82 ± 6. 11 (19-42)	.941
Gravidity (mean ± S.D.)	4.26 ± 2.25	2.27 ± 1.34	.105
Parity (mean ± S.D.)	2.00 ± 1.52	1.09 ± 1.22	.254
Abortions (mean ± S.D.)	1.26 ± 1.37	0.18 ± 0.40	.002[a]
Gestational age (mean ± S.D.)	31.71 ± 9.188	32.73 ± 10.59	.533
Previous cesarean section	27 (71.1%)	2 (18.2%)	.004[a]
Previous curettage	15 (39.5%)	1 (9.1%)	.076
≥2 Previous curettages	11 (22.4%)	0	.05[a]
Previous myomectomy	2 (5.3%)	0	1.000
Any previous procedure (c-section, curettage, or myomectomy)	30 (78.9%)	2 (18.2%)	<0.00r[a]
Placenta previa	19 (50.0%)	1 (9.1%)	.017[a]
% Remodeled vessels in full depth of uterine wall (mean ± S.D.)	23.23 ± 23.01	70.59 ± 33.19	.111
% Remodeled vessels in deep myometrium (mean ± S.D.)	6.14 ± 11.91	0	.002[a]
Cases with partially remodeled vessels	13 (34.2%)	0	<.001[a]
Maximal depth of remodeled vessels (mm; mean ± S.D.)	2.82 ± 1.54	1.80 ± 0.63	.001[a]
% Multinucleated interstitial trophoblasts (mean ± S.D.)	6.61 ± 6.61	5.91 ± 4.23	.147
Maximal depth of interstitial trophoblasts (mm; mean ± S.D.)	3.57 ± 2.02	2.63 ± 1.36	.009[a]

[a]Statistically significant.

Reprinted with permission from Tantbirojn P, Crum CP, Parast MM. Pathophysiology of placenta creta: the role of decidua and extravillous trophoblast. *Placenta.* 2008;29:639-645.

contrasted this to the creta cases which showed defective or only partial remodeling and hence lacking trophoblastic replacement.

Figure 4-6 demonstrates the various degrees of remodeling among creta patients. Figure 4-6A and B demonstrate creta cases with completely remodeled vessels. Figure 4-6C and D show partial remodeling, and Figure 4-6E and F demonstrate cases that completely lack vessel remodeling. The cytokeratin staining identifies the trophoblasts.

Placenta increta and percreta are associated with a dehiscence of the uterine scar therefore leading to chorionic villi being present deep within the uterine wall, hence the extravillous trophoblasts gain access to the deep myometrium.[30]

Others have discussed that perhaps absent or blocked proteases play a role.[36] As discussed in previous chapter, proteases assist in placental anchoring destruction

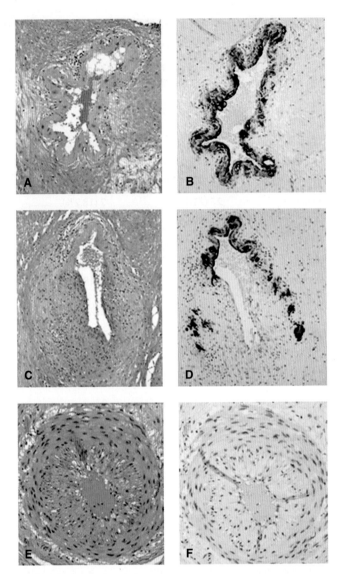

FIGURE 4-6   A-F, Original magnification ×100, E and F, original magnification ×200. A and B, Examples of creta with completely remodeled vessels. C and D, Examples of creta with partial remodeling. E and F, Examples of creta which completely lack vessel remodeling. The cytokeratin staining identifies the trophoblasts. (Reprinted with permission from Tantbirojn P, Crum CP, Parast MM. Pathophysiology of placenta creta: the role of decidua and extravillous trophoblast. *Placenta.* 2008;29:639-645.[30])

of vascular walls via endovascular nonvillous trophoblasts, therefore some degree of destruction exists.[30,36] However a faulty protease-antiprotease balance may cause abnormalities.[36]

Radiological Signs of Cretas

Radiological evaluation of cretas will be discussed in further detail in Chapter 5: Diagnostic imaging but briefly **the following are signs of cretas**[26]:

- absence of the hypoechoic space between the placenta and the myometrium
- vascular lacunae

- bridging vessels at the uterine-placenta or myometrial-bladder interface
- myometrial thickness behind the placenta of <1 mm
- bulging of the placenta through the myometrium and into adjacent tissues

Although cesarean scar pregnancies are a form of creta, we will discuss them separately.

Prior cesareans cause scarring in the lower uterine segment and can cause distorted anatomy. A common incidental finding on gynecologic ultrasounds in women with a prior cesarean is a uterine niche.

 PITFALL

The biggest concern regarding pregnancy in the presence of a uterine niche is that the niche can serve as an implantation site for an embryo, which can lead to complications and rarely results in a viable pregnancy.

UTERINE NICHE

Uterine niches have been reported in nearly 60% of patients with a history of cesarean and these niches can serve as site of implantation for the embryo leading to a cesarean scar ectopic.[37]

Several studies have focused on the characteristics of a uterine niche.[3,37] Niches have various appearances, but are a wedge-shaped, anechoic defect located in the anterior aspect of the myometrium in the lower uterine segment (Figure 4-7A and B).[25] Others describe the finding as a cystic lesion within the incision site.

Measurements of myometrial thickness at the location of the scar compared to the adjacent unaffected myometrium have been studied.[3] Ofili et al defined a 50% loss of myometrium as "severe deficiency."[3] The diagnosis according to Jurkovic et al. can be made with either a visible gap or the 50% difference.[2] The clinical significance of the depth of the niche and the associated strength has not been studied.[37] However researchers surmise a niche of 80% increases the risk of rupture.[37] Niches have been reported in nearly 60% of patients with a history of cesarean.[37]

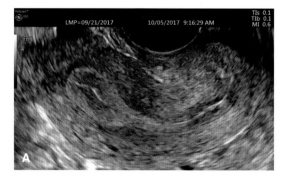
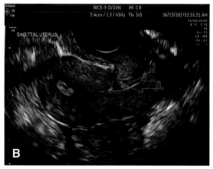

FIGURE 4-7 A, Normal anterior aspect of lower uterine segment. B, Presence of a cesarean scar niche.

One of the main risk factors for deficient scar is multiple cesareans, and the odds ratio doubles with each additional cesarean.[3] The biggest concern regarding pregnancy in the presence of a uterine niche is that the niche can serve as an implantation site for an embryo, which can lead to complications and rarely results in a viable pregnancy.

Uterine Niche Management

Pekar-Zlotin (2017) recommends against routine defective scar revision, stating that the utility and cost of the operations make them hard to justify and concluding that other complications could arise including poor scar healing, or adhesion formation, bleeding and potentially the need for hysterectomy, and the risk of uterine rupture still remains.[38] Therefore scar revision is not recommended at this time unless an usually large defect is discovered.[3]

CESAREAN SCAR PREGNANCY

The first case of CSP was reported by Solomon and Larsen in 1978.[39] The exact pathogenesis of a CSP is yet to be determined, and it is likely that many have gone undiagnosed over the years; however, the number diagnosed has continued to rise in the recent years. Current data show a CSP incidence of 1:1800 to 2226 (Figure 4-8).[40-42]

One study quoted 44% risk of miscarriage in cesarean scar pregnancies, and this would likely be higher if those with early concern for CSP were managed conservatively.[2]

Pekar-Zlotin et al found that over 50% of CSP had at least two prior cesareans.

Pathogenesis of Cesarean Scar Pregnancies

The exact cause has yet to be elucidated, however, several theories exist. It is thought that the blastocyte attaches to and begins invasion on the fibrous tissue at

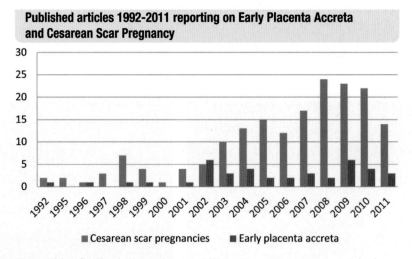

FIGURE 4-8 Number of early placenta accreta and cesarean scar pregnancy articles by year 1992 to 2011. (Reprinted with permission from Timor-Tritsch E. Early placenta accreta and Cesarean section scar pregnancy: a review. *J Obstet Gyncecol.* 2012.[43])

the wedge-shape myometrial defect, the niche, which is noted above and previously discussed.[4] Incomplete healing versus excessive fibrosis leads to the original defect in the lower uterine segment.[4] Vial et al have described two variations of CSP. One variation involves implantation of the amniotic sac directly in the scar site with subsequent progression of the pregnancy in the cervico-isthmus space and into the uterine cavity. The alternative is the result of deep implantation into the scar defect leading to rupture and bleeding during the first trimester.[44]

Godin hypothesized that a CSP occurs when implantation occurs through a microscopic dehiscent tract left behind by a previous scar.[45] Other researchers theorized through in vitro studies that areas of low oxygen tension, i.e., uterine scar, cause invading cytotrophoblasts to proliferate deep into the scar area.[43,46-48] Kliman also showed that trophoblasts prefer to attach to extracellular matrix over endometrial epithelial cells; hence the blastocyst favors scar tissue, which lacks epithelial cells.[48]

Ultrasound Diagnosis of Cesarean Scar Pregnancies

Diagnosing a CSP can be difficult, therefore, a full set of criteria has been established. Authors description includes an empty uterus and cervical canal, a clearly visible endometrium with absence of a pregnancy, and a gestational sac in the anterior aspect of the lower uterine segment surrounded by myometrium and fibrous tissue.[49,50] Timor-Tritsch developed a measurement system to assist in diagnosis of CSP (Figure 4-9A and B). He used transvaginal ultrasound to obtain a sagittal view of the uterus. Then he measured the uterine size by drawing a straight longitudinal line from the external cervical os to the fundus of the uterus. The midpoint of the line was determined, and this original line was transected by a perpendicular line, marking the middle of the uterine size. He then measured the distance from the external cervical os to the center of the gestational sac and the most distal point of the gestational sac and he found significant differences in these measurements (Table 4-6).

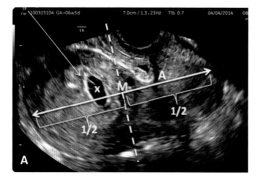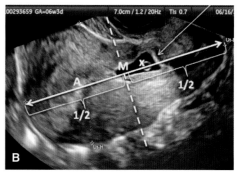

FIGURE 4-9 A and B, Using Timor-Tritsch method. A, Normally placed pregnancy, and B, abnormally placed pregnancy concerning for cesarean scan ectopic. (Reprinted with permission from Timor-Tritsch IE, Monteagudo A, Cali G, et al. Easy sonographic differential diagnosis between intrauterine pregnancy and cesarean delivery scar pregnancy in the early first trimester. *Am J Obstet Gynecol.* 2016;215:225.e1-225.e7.[51])

TABLE 4-6 Timor-Tritsch Measurement System Helps in Diagnosis of Cesarean Scar Pregnancy

Group	No. of Cases	Mean (SD) Distance From External Cervical Os to Center of Gestational Sac Relative to Midpoint of the Uterus, mm	Mean (SD) Distance From External Cervical Os to the Most Distant Point of the Gestational Sac Relative to the Midpoint of the Uterus, mm
Normal IUP	128	18.8 (6.9)	26.2 (7.3)
CSP	57	−10.6 (7.8)	−2.1 (6.7)
P-value		0.0001	0.0001

CSP, cesarean scar pregnancy; IUP, intrauterine pregnancy.

Modified and reprinted with permission from Timor-Tritsch IE, Monteagudo A, Cali G, et al. Easy sonographic differential diagnosis between intrauterine pregnancy and Cesarean delivery scar pregnancy in the early first trimester. *Am J Obstet Gynecol.* 2016;215:225.e1-225.e7.

Some authors have attempted to divide CSP into different classes. Shin Yu lin discussed Grades 1 to 4 (Figure 4-10).[52] The advancing gestational weeks increase the likelihood of a higher grade:

- **Grade 1**: Comprises a gestational sac that invades less than halfway through the anterior uterine wall thickness
- **Grade 2**: CSP invades more than halfway through the myometrial thickness
- **Grade 3**: Presence of a gestational sac and CSP bulging out anteriorly from the scar
- **Grade 4**: Presence of a richly vascularized mass at the site of the scar

Two types of cesarean scar ectopics have been defined:

- The first begins with deep implantation into the uterine scar, and growth progresses anteriorly, therefore leading to uterine rupture and hemorrhage (Figure 4-11).
- The second type involves implantation at the scar, however the pregnancy grows toward the uterine cavity or (Figure 4-11).

These pregnancies rarely make it to viability, however those that do, have an incredibly high risk for containing PAS.[25]

Differential Diagnosis of Cesarean Scar Pregnancy

When a vascular mass is seen in the lower aspect of the uterus, other diagnoses, some more common, must be considered. Differential diagnosis includes impending miscarriage, cervical ectopics, and adenomyosis. Cervical ectopics, also quite rare, are located within the cervical stroma but can be hard to differentiate from a CSP if the gestational sac is large.[25] The keys to determining the difference is location. Cervical ectopics are detected below the level of the internal os and may be implanted anteriorly, posteriorly, or laterally at the cervix. This is in contrast to a CSP which should always be anterior.[25] Adenomyosis is often ill-defined hypoechoic cysts that are small in size (2-3 mm) and their appearance often changes over the course of the menstrual cycle.[25] These women have a globular uterus and typically cyclic pain and pressure.

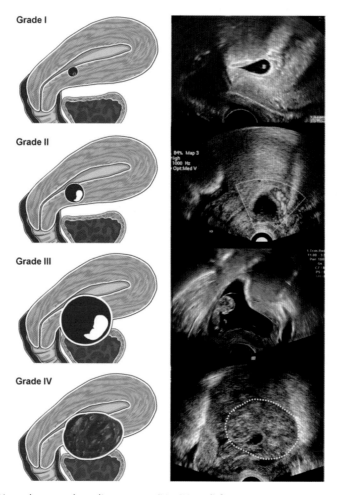

FIGURE 4-10 New ultrasound grading system (Lin SY et al) for cesarean scar pregnancy. (Reprinted with permission From Lin SY, Hsieh CJ, Tu YA et al. New ultrasound grading system for cesarean scar pregnancy and its implications for management strategies: an observational cohort study. *PLoS One*. 2018;13(8):e0202020. doi:10.1371/journal.pone.0202020.[52])

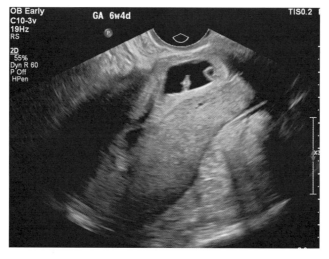

FIGURE 4-11 Cesarean scar ectopic identified on ultrasound.

REFERENCES

1. Martin JA, Hamilton BE, Osterman MJ, et al. Births: final data for 2016. *Natl Vital Stat Rep.* 2018;67:1.
2. Jurkovic D, Hillaby K, Woelfer B, et al. First trimester diagnosis and management of pregnancies implanted into the lower uterine segment cesarean section scar. *Ultrasound Obstet Gynecol.* 2003;21:220-227.
3. Ofili-Yebovi D, Ben-Nagi J, Sawyer E, et al. Deficient lower-segment cesarean section scars: prevalence and risk factors. *Ultrasound Obstet Gynecol.* 2008;31:72-77.
4. Singh D, Kaur L. When a Cesarean section scar is more that an innocent bystander in a subsequent pregnancy: ultrasound to the rescue. *J Clin Ultrasound.* 2017;45(6):319-327.
5. Miller DA, Chollet JA, Goodwin TM. Clinical risk factors for placenta praevia-placenta accreta. *Am J Obstet Gynecol.* 1997;177:210-214.
6. Zaideh SM, Abu-Heija AT, El-Jallad MF. Placenta praevia and accreta: analysis of a two-year experience. *Gynecol Obstet Investig.* 1998;46:96-98.
7. Bauer ST, Bonanno C. Abnormal placentation. *Semin Perinatol.* 2009;33(2):88-95.
8. Pridjian G, Rich NE, Montag AG. Pregnancy hemoperitoneum and placenta percreta in a patient with previous pelvic irradiation and ovarian failure. *Am J Obstet Gynecol.* 1990;162:1205-1206.
9. Norwitz ER, Stern HM, Grier H, et al. Placenta percreta and uterine rupture associated with prior whole body radiation therapy. *Obstet Gynecol.* 2001;98:929-931.
10. Van Thiel DH, Grodin JM, Ross GT, et al. Partial placenta accreta in pregnancies following chemotherapy for gestational trophoblastic neoplasms. *Am J Obstet Gynecol.* 1972;112:54-58.
11. Khong TY, Robertson WB. Placenta creta and placenta praevia creta. *Placenta.* 1987;8:399-409.
12. Khong TY. The pathology of placenta accreta, a worldwide epidemic. *J Clin Pathol.* 2008;61(12):611243-611246.
13. McKenna DA, Poder L, Goldman M, et al. Role of sonography in the recognition, assessment, and treatment of cesarean scar ectopic pregnancies. *J Ultrasound Med.* 2008;27:779.
14. Maymon R, Halperin R, Mendlovic S, et al. Ectopic pregnancies in a caesarean scar: review of the medical approach to an iatrogenic complication. *Hum Reprod Update.* 2004;10:515.
15. Seow KM, Huang LW, Lin YH, et al. Cesarean scar pregnancy: issues in management. *Ultrasound Obstet Gynecol.* 2004;23:247.
16. Alison M. Repair and regenerative process. In: O'Donnell Megee J, Isaacson PG, Wright NA, Dick HM, eds. *Oxford Textbook of Pathology. Vol. 1 Principles of Pathology.* New York: Oxford University Press; 1992:377-378.
17. Miller DA, Challet JA, Murphy TM. Clinical risk factors for placenta previa-placenta accreta. *Am J Obstet Gynecol.* 1997;177:210-214.
18. Downes KL, Hinkle SN, Sjaarda LA, et al. Previous prelabor or intrapartum cesarean delivery and risk of placenta previa. *Am J Obstet Gynecol.* 2015;212(669):e1-e6.
19. Son M, Grobman W. "Placental Disorders" Obstetric Evidence Based Guidelines. 3rd ed.; 2017:299-307.
20. Dashe JS, McIntire DD, Ramus RM, Santos-Ramos R, Twickler DM. Persistence of placenta previa according to gestational age at ultrasound detection. *Obstet Gynecol.* 2002;99:692-697.
21. Becker RH, Vonk R, Mende BC, Ragosch V, Entezami M. The relevance of placental location at 20-23 gestational weeks for prediction of placenta previa at delivery: evaluation of 8650 cases. *Ultrasound Obstet Gynecol.* 2001;17:496-501.
22. Oppenheimer L, Holmes P, Simpson N, Dabrowski A. Diagnosis of low-lying placenta: can migration in the third trimester predict outcome? *Ultrasound Obstet Gynecol.* 2001;18:100-102.
23. Spong CY, Mercer BM, D'alton M, et al. Timing of indicated late-preterm and early-term birth. *Obstet Gynecol.* 2011;118(2 Pt 1):323-333. doi:10.1097/AOG.0b013e3182255999.
24. Vergani P, Ornaghi S, Pozzi I, et al. Placenta previa: distance to internal os and mode of delivery. *Am J Obstet Gynecol.* 2009;201:266.e1-266.e5.
25. Woodward PJ, Kennedy A, Sohaey R, et al. *Diagnostic Imaging Obstetrics.* 3rd ed. Philadelphia: Elsevier; 2016:48-49, 800-805.
26. Moore TR. Placenta and umbilical cord imaging. In: *Creasy and Resnik's Maternal-Fetal Medicine: Principles and Practice.* 7th ed. Philadelphia: Elsevier; 2013;384-386.
27. Zelop CM, Harlow BL, Frigoletto FD, Safon LE, Saltzman DH. Emergency peripartum hysterectomy. *Am J Obstet Gynecol.* 1993;168:1443-1448.
28. Castaneda S, Karrison T, Ciblis LA. Peripartum hysterectomy. *J Perinat Med.* 2000;28:472-481.

29. Society for Maternal-Fetal Medicine. Quality of evidence: placenta accreta. *Am J Obstet Gynecol.* 2010;203:430-439.

30. Tantbirojn P, Crum CP, Parast MM. Pathophysiology of placenta creta: the role of decidua and extravillous trophoblast. *Placenta.* 2008;29:639-645.

31. Timor-Tritsch E, Monteagudo A, Cali G, et al. Cesarean scar pregnancy and early placenta accreta share common histology. *Ultrasound Obstet Gynecol.* 2014;43:383-395.

32. Jauniaex E, Collins S, Burton G. Placenta accreta spectrum: pathophysiology and evidence-based anatomy for prenatal ultrasound imaging. *Am J Obstet Gynecol.* 2018;218(1):75-87.

33. Baergen RN. *Manual of Benirschke and Kaufmann's Pathology of the Human Placenta.* New York: Springer-Verlag; 2005.

34. Blanc WA. Pathology of placenta accreta. *Verh Dtsch Ges Pathol.* 1976;60:393-399.

35. Benirschke K, Kaufmann K, Baergen P. *Pathology of the Human Placenta.* 5th ed. New York: Springer-Verlag; 2006.

36. Cramer SF, Heller DS. Placenta accreta and placenta increta: an approach to pathogenesis based on trophoblastic differentiation pathway. *Pediatr Dev Pathol.* 2016;19:320-333.

37. Regnard C, Nosbusch M, Fellemens C, et al. Cesarean section scar evaluation by saline contrast sonohysterogram. *Ultrasound Obstet Gynecol.* 2004;23(3):289-292.

38. Pekar-Zlotin M, Melcer Y, Levinsohn-Tavor O, et al. Cesarean scar pregnancy and morbidly adherent placenta: different or similar? *Isr Med Assoc J.* 2017;19(3):168-171.

39. Larsen JV, Solomon MH. Pregnancy in a uterine scar sacculus: an unusual cause of postabortal hemorrhage. A case report. *S Afr Med J.* 1978;53:142-143.

40. Ash A, Smith A, Maxwell D. Caesarean scar pregnancy. *Br J Obstet Gynaecol.* 2007;114:253.

41. Wang CB, Tseng CJ. Primary evacuation therapy for Cesarean scar pregnancy: three new cases and review. *Ultrasound Obstet Gynecol.* 2006;27:222.

42. Rosen T. Placenta accreta and cesarean scar pregnancy: overlooked costs of the rising cesarean section rate. *Clin Perinatol.* 2008;35:519.

43. Timor-Tritsch E, Monteagudo A. Unforeseen consequences of the increasing rate of cesarean deliveries: early placenta accreta and cesarean scar pregnancy. A review. *Am J Obstet Gynecol.* 2014;210(4):371-374.

44. Vial Y, Petignat P, Hohlfeld P. Pregnancy in a cesarean scar. *Ultrasound Obstet Gynecol.* 2000;16:592-593.

45. Godin PA, Bassil S, Donnez J. An ectopic pregnancy developing in a previous cesarean section scar. *Fertil Steril.* 1997;67:398-400.

46. Genbacev O, Zhou Y, Ludlow JW, Fisher SJ. Regulation of human placental development by oxygen tension. *Science.* 1997;277:1669-1672.

47. Norwitz ER. Defective implantation and placentation: laying the blueprint for pregnancy complications. *Reprod Biomed Online.* 2006;13:591-599.

48. Kliman HJ, Feinberg RF, Haimowitz JE. Human trophoblast-endometrial interactions in an in vitro suspension culture system. *Placenta.* 1990;11:349-367.

49. Maymon R, Halperin R, Mendlovic S, et al. Ectopic pregnancies in cesarean section scars: the 8 year experience of one medical center. *Hum Reprod.* 2004;19:278-284.

50. Osborn DA, Williams TR, Craig BM. Cesarean scar pregnancy: sonographic and magnetic resonance imaging findings, complications, and treatment. *J Ultrasound Med.* 2012;31:1449-1456.

51. Timor-Tritsch IE, Monteagudo A, Cali G, et al. Easy sonographic differential diagnosis between intrauterine pregnancy and Cesarean delivery scar pregnancy in the early first trimester. *Am J Obstet Gynecol.* 2016;215:225.e1-225.e7.

52. Lin S-Y, Hsieh C-J, Tu Y-A, et al. New ultrasound grading system for cesarean scar pregnancy and its implications for management strategies: an observational cohort study. *PLoS One.* 2018;13(8):e0202020. doi:10.1371/journal.pone.0202020.

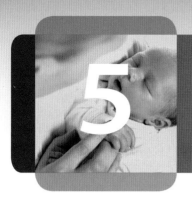

Diagnostic Imaging in Abnormal Placentation

Kimberly Vickers, Erin H. Burnett

INTRODUCTION AND RESEARCH

Placenta accreta spectrum (PAS) and abnormally invasive placenta (AIP) are the general terms used for placenta accreta. The varying forms of placenta accreta (Figure 5-1) range from a mild form known as accreta, to a more invasive form known as increta, and finally to the most invasive form known as percreta.[1] Accreta occurs when the placental villi attach to the myometrium rather than the decidua. In placenta increta, the villi penetrate into the myometrium. Percreta is characterized by chorionic villi attaching through the myometrium and possibly to adjacent structures. The most common site of attachment is the bladder. It may also attach to the rectum and occasionally to the bowel, although this is rare.

Two studies conducted in 1997 and 2005 included a total of 138 histologically confirmed abnormally implanted placentas. Based on the hysterectomy specimens, the types and frequency were accreta 79%, increta 14%, and percreta 7% (Figure 5-1).[1-3]

The exact pathogenesis for placenta accreta is not exactly known, but it is largely believed that many of the cases are a result of postoperative scarring. Theories for this have been supported by the observations that 80% of cases were associated with a history of previous cesarean delivery, curettage, and/or myomectomy.[4] The most common theories for the pathogenesis are related to abnormal vascularization resulting from the scarring process following surgery. Localized hypoxia in this scarred area may lead to both defective decidualization and excessive trophoblastic invasion. As a result, the placenta attaches directly to the myometrium.

In cases of partial or complete dehiscence of the uterine scar, the extravillous trophoblasts have access to the deeper parts of the myometrium, bladder serosa, and potentially beyond resulting in increta and percreta.

INCIDENCE

The incidence of PAS has increased significantly through the years. In the 1950s, abnormal placental attachment was 1 in 30,000 deliveries in the United States and only 1 in 10,000 deliveries in the 1960s. The current overall incidence of placenta accreta is 3 in 1000 deliveries. There has been a considerable increase over the past several decades, mainly due to the increased numbers of cesarean deliveries and multiple repeat cesareans.

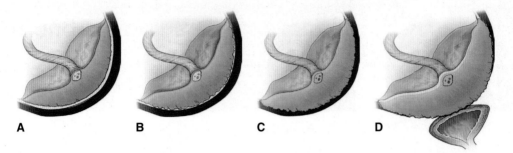

FIGURE 5-1 Types of placentation. A, Normal placentation. B, Accreta. C, Increta. D, Percreta.[1]

The rates of cesarean deliveries in the United States have increased from 2% in the 1950s to 5.8% in the 1970s. The rate from 2017 in the United States ranges from 22.5% to 37.8% across the country based on numbers from the National Center for Health Statistics.[5]

The rates of cesarean section vary widely per country. In 2016, the World Health Organization addressed the high rates of cesarean sections in Greece stating that over half of the deliveries in that country are by cesarean. This is between 50% and 70% with a large rate disparity between the public and private hospitals.[6] In Brazil, the cesarean rate is 55.6%. The country is currently trying to reverse the growing numbers. The United States is also trying to reduce the number of cesarean sections. The lowest rate of elective cesarean deliveries is in Finland with a rate of 6.6%, which is well below the World Health Organization's recommendation of 10% to 15%.[7]

ASSESSING FOR ABNORMAL PLACENTATION

Assessing for abnormally adherent placenta is similar to putting the pieces of a puzzle together. Assessment requires thorough medical history, maternal serum screening, and ultrasound. If the ultrasound shows sign of accreta, a magnetic resonance imaging (MRI) may be considered as a possible adjunctive tool, although, no single modality determines accreta with 100% accuracy. The final diagnosis of accreta is based on the results of a histology of specimen (Figures 5-2 to 5-4).

RISK FACTORS FOR PAS AND SCREENING TO PREDICT WHO MAY BE AT RISK

A multitude of risk factors for accreta exist. Thorough documentation of all factors is important.

- The biggest risk factor is a history of uterine surgery, to include but not limited to, cesarean section, myomectomy, intrauterine adhesion removal, dilation and curettage, ectopic pregnancy, cornual resection, and endometrial ablation.
- Other risk factors include pelvic irradiation, advanced maternal age, Asherman syndrome, grand multiparity, hypertensive disorders, and smoking.

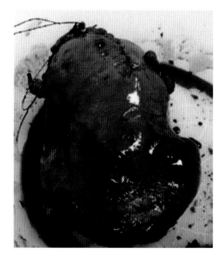

FIGURE 5-2 Uterus after cesarean hysterectomy performed at 34 weeks. Specimen includes uterus with placenta percreta, which had bladder invasion.

- In vitro fertilization (IVF) procedures also contribute to accretas. This is related to the IVF stimulation protocols. Studies have shown that IVF induces morphological and structural changes and can disrupt the expression of relevant genes in the endometrium. These changes could contribute to abnormal implantation.[8]
- The most important concerning combination of risk factors for accreta is placenta previa with a history of prior cesarean section (Table 5-1). In a prospective study, the frequency of accreta increased in proportion with the growing number of cesarean deliveries. Previa at the time of their first cesarean, the risk was 3%, but this risk dramatically increases. Current previa with current cesarean being their third increases the risk of accrete to 40% and a mother having her five or more cesarean has a 67% risk of accreta.[9]

- Serum screening used to assess for aneuploidy risk in pregnancy has been associated with adverse outcomes, such as preeclampsia and intrauterine growth restriction. Both of these are thought to be diseases of abnormal trophoblastic invasion. Studies have shown an association between placenta accreta and elevated msAFP and fbHCG in second trimester maternal serum screening.[10,11] If placenta accreta develops in the first trimester and there is a disruption of the maternal-placental barrier, it would correlate with an alteration of PAPP-A levels.
- Mothers who have had an elevated msAFP of >2 or 2.5 MoM have also been associated with AIP. An elevated msAFP can support an ultrasound-based diagnosis of accreta. The elevated msAFP alone is an inconsistent finding and is not useful by itself for diagnosis. In addition, a normal msAFP does not exclude the diagnosis of accreta.

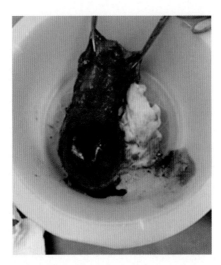

FIGURE 5-3 Uterus after cesarean hysterectomy performed at 29 weeks due to preeclampsia with severe features and vaginal bleeding. Noted to have placenta increta.

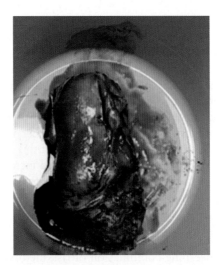

FIGURE 5-4 Uterus after hysterectomy with fetus in situ performed at 18 weeks due to prelabor premature rupture of membranes and vaginal bleeding. Suspected and confirmed cesarean scar ectopic with placenta percreta confirmed on pathology.

TABLE 5-1 Risk of Accreta Based on Presence or Absence of Placenta Previa and the Number of Cesareans

Cesarean Number	Placenta previa	No previa
First (primary)	3.3	0.03
Second	11	0.2
Third	40	0.1
Fourth	61	0.8
Fifth	67	0.8
Sixth or more	67	4.7

Modified with permission from Society for Maternal Fetal Medicine: Quality of evidence: placenta accreta. *Am J Obstet Gynecol.* 2010;203:430-439.

ULTRASOUND: PRIMARY DIAGNOSTIC TOOL

In pregnancy, ultrasound is the primary modality of choice to assess not only the fetus, but the placenta as well. This method is inexpensive and noninvasive. There are multiple uses of ultrasound to further assess in the diagnosis of abnormally adherent placenta. In conjunction with normal 2D ultrasound, color flow Doppler and 3D power Doppler with multislice viewing can add additional layers to help increase the confidence in the diagnosis.

The best imaging method is high-frequency transvaginal ultrasound because it improves the near-field resolution interface between the placenta and lower uterine segment. This is especially helpful in cases of placenta previa or posterior placenta. Ideally, placenta accreta is first suspected because of findings on ultrasound when the patient is asymptomatic.

Authors reported that ultrasound is a useful tool to diagnosis accreta with a 77% to 93% sensitivity and a 71% to 98% specificity.[12] Studies have also shown that the prevalence of ultrasound findings suggestive of accrete changes throughout the pregnancy.

Assessment of the Site of Implantation

First-Trimester Ultrasound

First-trimester ultrasound is important, especially in mothers with a history of a previous cesarean. An early first-trimester ultrasound at 6 to 9 weeks gestational age allows for early assessment of implantation to evaluate for normal (Figure 5-5A) versus low implantation/cesarean scar pregnancy (CSP) (Figure 5-5B). Timor-Tritsch developed a measurement system to assist in diagnosis of CSPs (Table 5-2).[13] He used transvaginal ultrasound to obtain a sagittal view of the uterus. Then he measured the uterine size by drawing a straight longitudinal line from the external cervical os to the fundus of the uterus. The midpoint of the line was determined and this original line was transected by a perpendicular line, marking the middle of the uterine size. He then measured the distance from the external cervical os to the center of the gestational sac and the most distal point of the gestational sac and he found significant differences in these measurements.

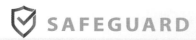 **SAFEGUARD**

> First-trimester ultrasound is important, especially in mothers with a history of a previous cesarean. An early first-trimester ultrasound at 6 to 9 weeks gestational age allows for early assessment of implantation to evaluate for normal versus low implantation/cesarean scar pregnancy

A panoramic, longitudinal, sagittal scan can be used to determine the location of the gestational sac. Divide the uterus in half with an imaginary line. If the gestational sac is above the line, it is most likely a normal implantation. If the gestational sac is below it, suspect a CSP or a cervical pregnancy and hence high risk of accreta.

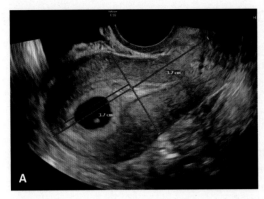 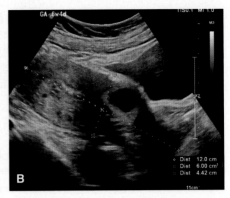

FIGURE 5-5 A and B, Measurements using Timor-Tristch method of comparative distance from the external cervical os to the gestational sac relative to midpoint of uterus between normal intrauterine pregnancies (A) and abnormal placentation, i.e., cesarean scar pregnancies (B).

It is hypothesized that cesarean scar pregnancy and accreta are not separate entities but a continuum of the same condition. A cesarean scar pregnancy is a precursor to accreta.[13]

 SAFEGUARD

It is hypothesized that cesarean scar pregnancy and accreta are not separate entities but a continuum of the same condition. A cesarean scar pregnancy is a precursor to accreta.[13]

Findings of Ultrasound at 11 to 14 weeks

Additional signs of adherent placenta can be seen at 11 to 14 weeks. Prevalence does increase with advancing gestational age. Multiple ultrasound findings can be seen in order to assist with the diagnosis of abnormally adherent placenta which include:

- loss of placental homogenicity
- loss of normal clear space
- retroplacental myometrial thinning
- disruption of bladder wall-uterine serosa interface
- placental bulging into the bladder wall
- exophytic mass

TABLE 5-2   Timor-Tritsch Measurement assists in Diagnosis of Cesarean Scar Pregnancy

Group	No. of Cases	Mean (SD) Distance From External Cervical Os to Center of Gestational Sac Relative to Midpoint of the Uterus, mm	Mean (SD) Distance From External Cervical Os to the Most Distant Point of the Gestational Sac Relative to the Midpoint of the Uterus, mm
Normal IUP	128	18.8 (6.9)	26.2 (7.3)
CSP	57	−10.6 (7.8)	−2.1 (6.7)
P-value		0.0001	0.0001

CSP, cesarean scar pregnancy; IUP, intrauterine pregnancy.

Modified with permission from Timor-Tritsch IE, Monteagudo A, Cali G, et al. Easy sonographic differential diagnosis between intrauterine pregnancy and cesarean delivery scar pregnancy in the early first trimester. *Am J Obstet Gynecol.* 2016;215(2):225.e1-225.e7.

Loss of Homogenicity

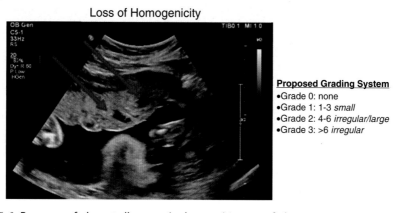

Proposed Grading System
•Grade 0: none
•Grade 1: 1-3 *small*
•Grade 2: 4-6 *irregular/large*
•Grade 3: >6 *irregular*

FIGURE 5-6 Presence of placenta llacunae (red arrows) in case of placenta accrete using grading scale. (Reprinted with permission from Finberg H, Williams J. Placenta accreta: prospective sonographic diagnosis in patients with placenta previa and prior cesarean section. *J Ultrasound Med.* 1992;11(7):333-343.)

Loss of Homogenicity

The placenta will lose its normal smooth echotexture due to multiple intraplacental sonolucent spaces called *placental lacunae*. This will give the placenta a "Swiss cheese" or "moth eaten" appearance (Figure 5-6). A proposed grading scale of the sonolucent areas states that the presence of multiple abnormal lacunae is the best studied and most useful 2D sonographic marker. Findings have been correlated with a detection rate of 100% for accreta especially when the following findings are observed:

• loss of clear space
• retroplacental myometrial thinning
• disruption of the bladder wall-uterine serosa interface and placental bulging into the bladder wall
• exophytic mass

DIAGNOSIS OF ACCRETA WITH THE FOLLOWING FINDINGS

• loss of clear space
• retroplacental myometrial thinning
• disruption of the bladder wall-uterine serosa interface and placental bulging into the bladder wall
• exophytic mass

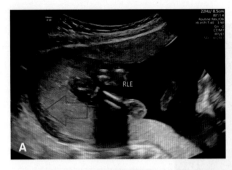
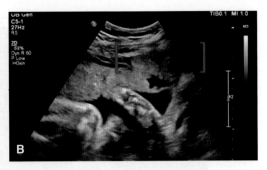

FIGURE 5-7 A, Normal clear space (red arrow) present in normal placentation. B, Loss of normal clear (red parenthesis) in abnormal placentation.

Video 5-1 Loss of normal clear.

Loss of Clear Space

Loss of normal clear space refers to the absence of the normal hypoechoic area behind the placenta (Figure 5-7). This finding may be angle dependent and can be absent in normal anterior placentas. Due to the false positive rate, this should not be the sole ultrasound marker used for diagnosis.

Retroplacental Myometrial Thinning

Retroplacental myometrial thinning is a measurement of <1 mm of the clear space posterior to the placenta (Figure 5-8) and is suggestive of adherent placenta. This progressive thinning indicates the proximity of the placental tissue to the peritoneal serosa and surrounding viscera, mainly the bladder.[15]

Disruption of Bladder Wall-Uterine Serosa Interface and Placental Bulging Into the Bladder Wall

The loss or disruption of the normally continuous white line representing the bladder wall-uterine serosa interface (Figure 5-9) may be more consistent with greater compromise due to placental increta or percreta. This may sometimes be difficult to differentiate between bladder wall irregularities and accreta.[16]

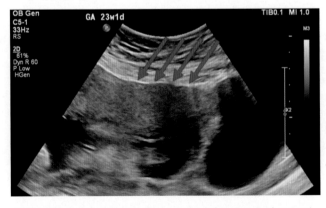

FIGURE 5-8 Retroplacental myometrial thinning (red arrows).

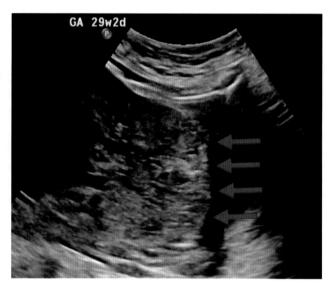

FIGURE 5-9 Example depicting the bladder wall-uterine surface interface (red arrows).

Bulging of the placenta into the posterior wall of the bladder suggests invasion of the uterine wall and possible attachment to the uterine serosa and potentially the bladder (Figure 5-10).

Exophytic Mass

An exophytic mass is when there is disruption of the uterine serosa-bladder wall creating an abnormal bulge of placental tissue into the adjacent structures, mainly the bladder (Figure 5-11).

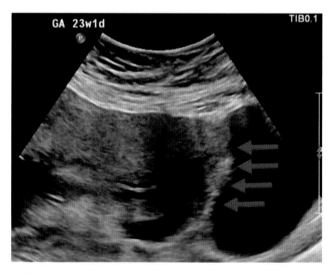

FIGURE 5-10 Placenta noted on ultrasound to be bulging into the bladder (red arrows).

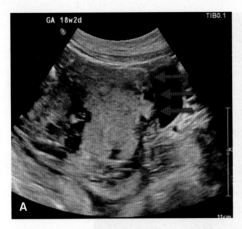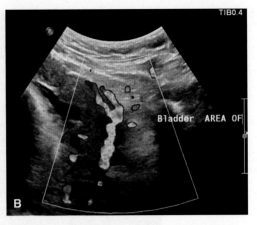

FIGURE 5-11 A, Exophytic mass originating from the placenta (red arrows) noted to be invading other areas. B, Exophytic mass with color flow.

CONFIRMING WITH USE OF COLOR FLOW DOPPLER

Color flow Doppler is a valuable tool in confirming the diagnosis of accreta when used in conjunction with other ultrasound findings. Out of all the different ultrasound findings, abnormal vasculature on color flow Doppler has the best combination of sensitivity and specificity in the prediction of invasive placentation.

There are five color flow Doppler signs:

Video 5-2
Subplacental hypervascularity.

- subplacental hypervascularity, (Figure 5-12)
- uterovesical hypervascularity,
- bridging vessels,
- feeder vessels,
- lacunar turbulent flow

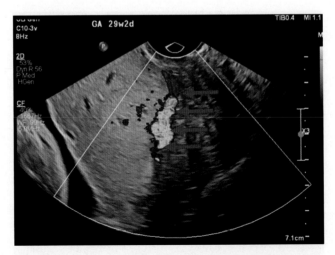

FIGURE 5-12 In subplacental hypervascularity you will see a Doppler (red arrows) signal in the placental bed. This flow will be multidirectional and demonstrate aliasing.

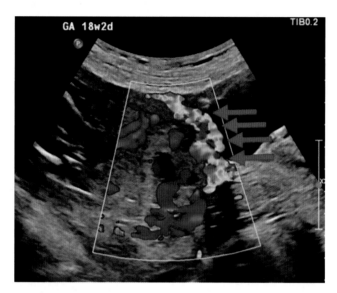

FIGURE 5-13 Uterovesicular hypervascularity (red arrows).

Uterovesical Hypervascularity

Uterovesical hypervascularity, the Doppler signal, between the uterus and bladder will be multidirectional in flow and demonstrate aliasing (distortion) (see Figure 5-13).

Bridging Vessels

Bridging vessels are vessels that appear to extend in perpendicular fashion from the placenta into the bladder serosa (Figure 5-14).

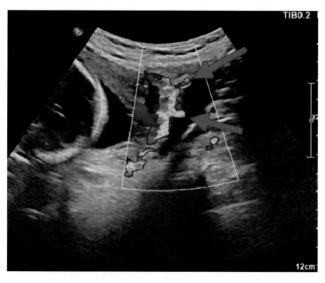

FIGURE 5-14 Arrows identifying bridging vessels.

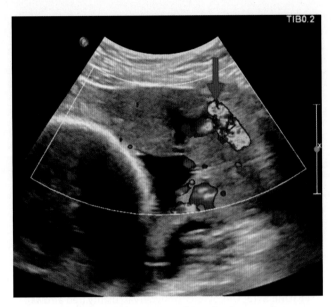

FIGURE 5-15 Arrow identifying feeder vessels.

Feeder Vessels

Feeder vessels are large vessels that extend from the placental bed into the placenta with turbulent entry into the llacunae (Figure 5-15).

Lacunar Turbulent Flow

Lacunar turbulent flow is noted in the lacunae with a "thunderstorm" like appearance (Figure 5-16). The lacunae can have a pulsatile flow of >10 cm/s.

Although not one of the five color flow Doppler signs, turbulent flow within the cervix is a marker for postpartum hemorrhage and can be associated with adherent placenta (Figure 5-17).

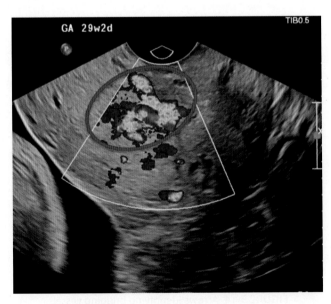

FIGURE 5-16 Turbulent flow (circled).

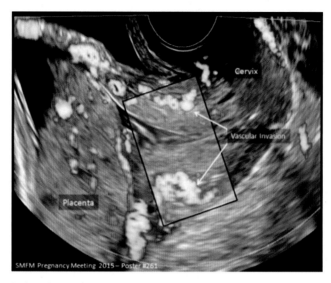

FIGURE 5-17 Turbulent flow within cervical stroma suggesting invasion and a risk factor for postpartum hemorrhage.[18]

UTILIZING 3D ULTRASOUND IMAGING

Three-dimensional (3D) power Doppler allows multiplane imaging display in the sagittal, coronal, and axial planes at the same time. Power Doppler added to the 3D viewing planes allows images of the vasculature to be manipulated and allows identification of vessels invading the bladder. Three-dimensional ultrasound can be used as an adjunctive tool with 2D. With the 3D power Doppler, it can be used to differentiate between placenta accreta and percreta. The lateral view is used to observe the intraplacental vasculature and serosa-bladder complex along the sagittal axis of the maternal pelvis. The basal view is used to illustrate the serosa-bladder wall interface in a 90° rotation of the lateral view (Figures 5-18 and 5-19).

3D power Doppler is effective in identifying intraplacental hypervascularity, inseparable cotyledonal, intervillous circulations, and tortuous vascularity with "chaotic branching." Tortuous vascularity with chaotic branching is when vessels grow in an irregular manner in a tortuous course, varying in calibers and complex vessel arrangements. This is seen in tumoral vessels of ovarian malignancies.

3D power Doppler is also useful in evaluating normal placental vasculature. In a basal view of a normal placenta, the vessels in the uterine serosa-bladder border will be discretely arranged. The cotyledonal and the intervillous circulation will be separately distributed. The cotyledonal circulation is longer and more apparent than the intervillous circulation (Figure 5-20).[17]

3D Multislice View Doppler

A majority of newer ultrasound systems have 3D ability and the capability to save 3D volumes. These can then later be manipulated and a multislice program can be

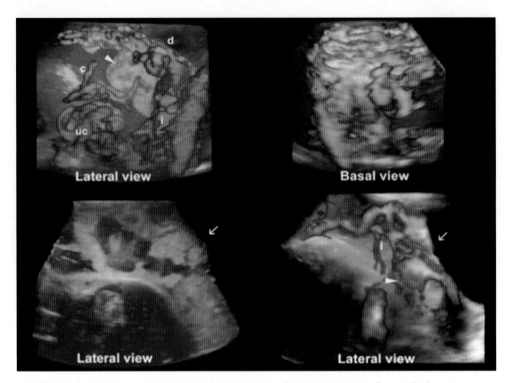

FIGURE 5-18 3D images of the lateral and basal view of the placenta interface with the uterus and bladder. Arrows indicate exophytic placenta; arrowheads indicate aneurysm. c, cotyledonal circulation; d, decidual plate; i, intervillous circulation; uc, umbilical cord. (Shih J-C. Role of three-dimensional power Doppler in the antenatal diagnosis of placenta accreta: comparison with gray-scale and color Doppler techniques. *Ultrasound Obstet Gynecol.* 2009;33(2):193-203.)

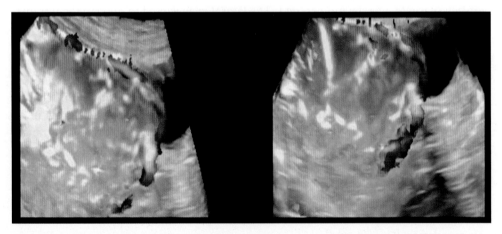

FIGURE 5-19 3D depiction of the serosa-bladder wall interface. (Shih J-C. Role of three-dimensional power Doppler in the antenatal diagnosis of placenta accreta: comparison with gray-scale and color Doppler techniques. *Ultrasound Obstet Gynecol.* 2009;33(2):193-203.)

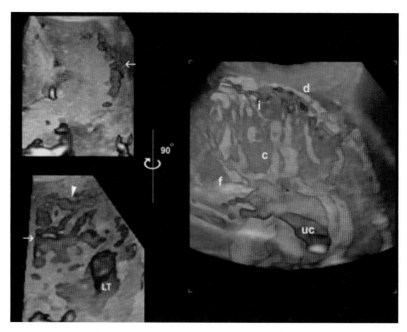

FIGURE 5-20 3D power doppler in normal placentation. The arrows indicate the same group of vessels; arrowhead indicates a group of discretely distributed vessels. c, cotyledonal circulation; d, decidual plate; f, fetal (chorionic) plate; i, intervillous circulation; LT, left uterine artery; uc, umbilical cord. (Shih J-C. Role of three-dimensional power Doppler in the antenatal diagnosis of placenta accreta: comparison with gray-scale and color Doppler techniques. *Ultrasound Obstet Gynecol.* 2009;33(2):193-203.)

employed. Precision slicing of the data can be controlled by the user and can vary from 0 to 1 mm in thickness up to potentially 16 mm in thickness. This gives the ability to use the ultrasound information to display a study similar to an MRI. The user can adjust the slice interval spacing and select how many views to display depending on the program. Depending on the program, the display can view 4, 9, 16, or up to 25 2D slices at one time. The user will have the ability to rotate the multiplanar view. Unlike MRI, the slices are instantly updated to reflect a new perspective (Figures 5-21 to 5-23).

The sonographic findings using 3D multislice view (MSV) Doppler to evaluate accuracy of the diagnosis of abnormally adherent placenta were compared to the intraoperative findings and histological results from the removed uteri in the cases of emergent hysterectomy. It was found that 3D MSV Doppler increased the accuracy and predictive values of the diagnostic criteria in comparison with 3D power Doppler.

When using 3D MSV Doppler to assess crowded vessels over the peripheral subplacental zone to detect for difficult placental separation and considerable intraoperative blood loss in cases of AIP, the sensitivity and negative predictive

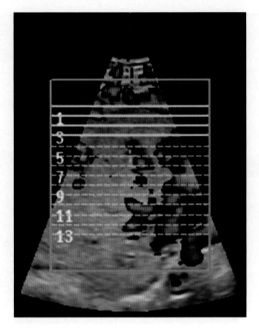

FIGURE 5-21 3D multiple slice views obtainable at various levels to improve diagnosis.

value increased from 79.6% and 82.2% to 82.6% and 84%, respectively. In cases of disruption of the uterine serosa-bladder interface when assessing for AIP, the sensitivity, specificity, and positive predictive value were 90.9%, 68.8%, and 47%, respectively. Using the 3D MSV Doppler, this was increased to 100%, 71.8%, and 50%, respectively.[12]

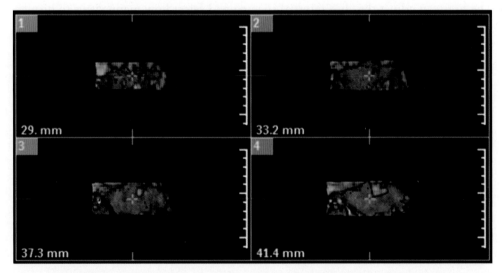

FIGURE 5-22 Various views can be compared to look and identify level of invasion.

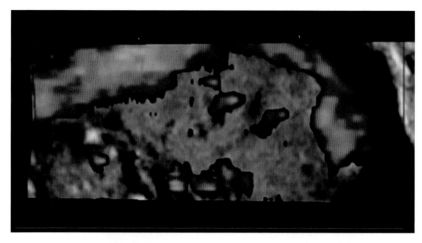

FIGURE 5-23 Images can be zoomed-in to obtain better views.

MAGNETIC RESONANCE IMAGING

Magnetic resonance imaging (MRI) is a helpful tool in conjunction with ultrasound in cases of suspected placental invasion or bladder involvement observed on ultrasound. MRI is also helpful in evaluating posterior placenta or if the ultrasound is inconclusive. MRI to assess for AIP is done without gadolinium contrast, which can cross the placenta into the fetal circulation to be excreted by the fetal kidneys into the amniotic fluid. The effects of gadolinium-based contrast on a developing fetus are unknown. Although gadolinium may improve the diagnostic performance, it is generally avoided in pregnancy. The US Food and Drug Administration classifies gadolinium as a Class C drug and should be used only if the potential benefits outweigh the potential risk to the fetus.[19]

The European Society of Urogenital Radiology Contrast Media Safety Committee guidelines state that the highest risk gadolinium contrast media are contraindicated in pregnant women, while the intermediate and lowest risk gadolinium contrast media may be given in the lowest dose required to provide essential diagnostic information.[20]

The recommended gestational age for MRI to evaluate for placenta accreta is 24 to 30 weeks. The normal placenta exhibits homogenous intermediate signal and is usually clearly distinct from the myometrium, which is more heterogeneous and hyperintense. Before 24 weeks, the placenta is immature and MRI performs poorly in diagnosing abnormal placentation. After 30 weeks, the internal placental signal becomes more heterogeneous as the placenta matures and therefore identifying the interfaces becomes difficult and detection of abnormal placentation is compromised.

The features seen in placenta accreta, such as lumpy contour, rounded edges, uterine bulging, and placenta previa, result from the tethering that hinders the normal migration of the placenta during gestation.

As in ultrasound, MRI demonstrates multiple findings suggestive of AIP. These findings include:

- uterine bulging into the bladder
- heterogeneous signal of intensity within the placenta

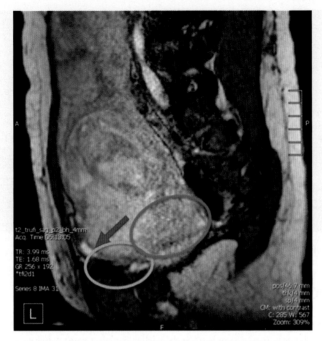

FIGURE 5-24 Red arrow depicts uterine bulging into the bladder, blue circle represents heterogeneous signal of intensity within the placenta, white circle identifies the focal interruption of the myometrium.

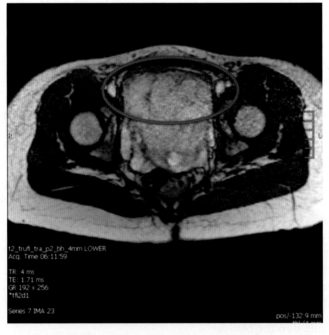

FIGURE 5-25 Intraplacental bands identified.

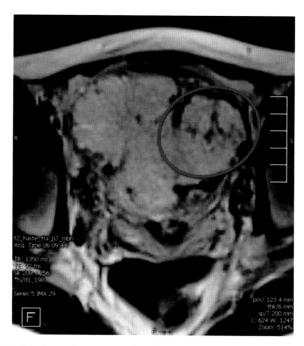

FIGURE 5-26 Area of concern within the placenta for abnormal vascularity.

- presence of dark intraplacental bands on the T2-weighted imaging, abnormal placental vascularity
- focal interruption of the myometrium
- tenting of the bladder and direct visualization of the invasion of the pelvis structures by the placental tissue

The most sensitive feature followed by marked heterogenicity of the placenta was dark intraplacental bands on the T2-weighted sequences (Figures 5-24 to 5-26). The sensitivity, specificity, positive predictive value, and negative predictive value of MRI in predicting placenta accreta derived from three studies were, respectively, 88.89%-100%, 100%, 100%, and 92.86%-100%.[21]

SUMMARY

It should be noted that no single diagnostic modality determines the placental invasiveness with absolute accuracy. Ultrasound, as well as MRI, has positives and negatives in assessment mainly related to the cost of each, maternal habitus for both modalities, gestational age, and need for stillness and breath holding for MRI.

Color flow Doppler remains the primary mode for antenatal diagnosis with MRI reserved for cases where ultrasound is inconclusive. Color flow Doppler ultrasound and MRI have nearly the same sensitivity for the diagnosis of AIP. Both of these modalities have complimentary roles in cases of inconclusive findings. When imaging with one modality is difficult, the other modality may be useful in obtaining the diagnosis.

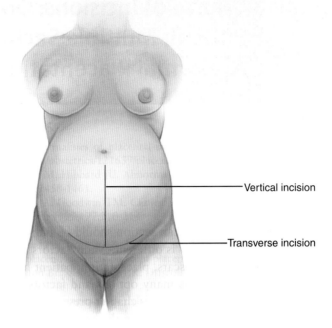

FIGURE 6-1 Types of abdominal incisions used for cesarean delivery: vertical or low transverse. The transverse incision is the most commonly used incision for cesarean section in the United States. The vertical incision is often used in cases of emergent cesarean sections, known multiple prior surgeries, or preexisting vertical skin incision. (With permission from Hatfield NT. *Introductory Maternity and Pediatric Nursing*. 3rd ed. Philadelphia: Wolters Kluwer; 2014.)

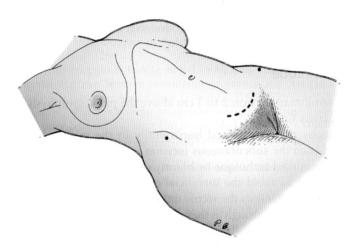

FIGURE 6-2 Skin incision for Pfannenstiel technique. A semilunar skin incision approximately 2 cm above the pubic symphysis is made. The direction of the incision should aim toward the anterior superior iliac spines. (Reprinted with permission from Jones HW, Rock JA. *Te Linde's Operative Gynecology*. 11th ed. Wolters Kluwer; 2015.)

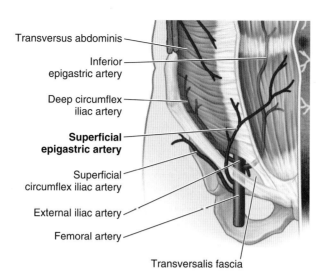

Transversus abdominis

Inferior epigastric artery

Deep circumflex iliac artery

Superficial epigastric artery

Superficial circumflex iliac artery

External iliac artery

Femoral artery

Transversalis fascia

FIGURE 6-3 The superficial epigastric vessels run in the lateral subcutaneous tissue just lateral to the rectus muscles. Care must be taken to avoid the superficial epigastric vessels which are often cut or torn during Pfannenstiel incisions. (Reprinted with permission from Agur AM, Dalley AF. *Grant's Atlas of Anatomy*. 14th ed. Philadelphia: Wolters Kluwer; 2017.)

- Any perforating vessels encountered should be individually cauterized. If they retract without being properly cauterized, a postoperative rectus hematoma can develop.
- The rectus muscles are then separated in the midline and lateralized (Figure 6-6).
- The peritoneum is identified at the most cephalad point and entered sharply.
- The peritoneal incision is then extended with care taken to avoid the bladder. A modified technique is to enter the peritoneum and extend the opening bluntly.

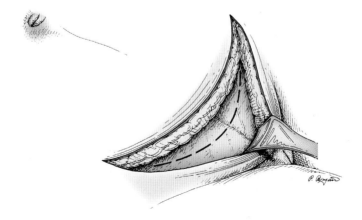

FIGURE 6-4 Fascial incision for a Pfannenstiel incision. The fascia is cut in a semilunar fashion similar to the skin incision. The lateral edges of the incision can be extended past the length of the skin incision to gain more exposure. (Reprinted with permission from Jones HW, Rock JA. *Te Linde's Operative Gynecology*. 11th ed. Wolters Kluwer; 2015.)

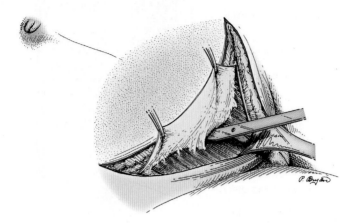

FIGURE 6-5 Elevating the fascia from the rectus muscle during Pfannenstiel technique. Identify and cauterize the perforating vessels before cutting them to avoid hematoma. (Reprinted with permission from Jones HW, Rock JA. *Te Linde's Operative Gynecology*. 11th ed. Wolters Kluwer; 2015.)

Joel-Cohen Low Transverse Abdominal Entry

Another common low transverse abdominal entry used during cesarean section is the Joel-Cohen method. In a Cochrane review, the Joel-Cohen incision was found to be associated with less fever, pain and analgesic requirements, less blood loss, and shorter duration of surgery and hospital stay than the Pfannenstiel method.[2] The Joel-Cohen low transverse technique can be useful in performing stat cesarean sections as the abdomen can be entered in seconds by an experienced obstetrician. In addition, there is a decreased chance of accidentally severing the superficial epigastric vessels and rectus perforating vessels.

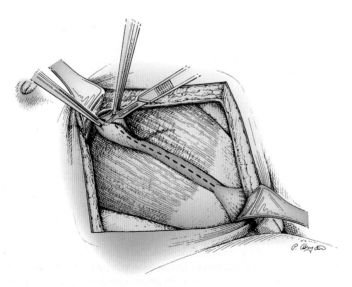

FIGURE 6-6 Dividing the rectus muscles during Pfannenstiel technique. If there is scaring, the rectus muscles may need to be sharply divided. (Reprinted with permission from Jones HW, Rock JA. *Te Linde's Operative Gynecology*. 11th ed. Wolters Kluwer; 2015.)

Technique for Joel-Cohen Low Transverse Abdominal Entry

- This incision is 1 to 2 cm more cephalad than the Pfannenstiel incision and is linear as opposed to curvilinear.
- The subcutaneous tissue is incised horizontally in the midline to expose the fascia, and then a small horizontal incision is made in the fascia to expose the rectus muscles.
- The rectus muscles are separated bluntly by manual traction in a craniocaudal direction, then in a lateral direction.
- The peritoneum is entered and extended bluntly.

Complications of Low Transverse Abdominal Incision

- Poor exposure if complications arise or access needed outside of the pelvis

    Low transverse incisions are usually adequate for exposure for the majority of cesarean sections. However, they give very poor exposure for complications outside of the pelvis. If a fundal uterine incision is needed due to placentation, fetal position or scarring, the fundus will likely be inaccessible and the skin incision will need to be extended. If adhesive disease involving the bowel is present, mobilization and evaluation will be difficult.[1]

- Superficial epigastric vessels are often encountered and can be incidentally cut or torn during the procedure. If this occurs, the epigastric vessels often retract into the subcutaneous tissue and must be dissected and cauterized or tied to avoid hematomas and extensive blood loss.

Midline Vertical Abdominal Incision

Midline vertical abdominal incision has many advantages. It is quick and relatively bloodless when doing a stat cesarean section or with a patient with coagulation defects. This incision allows adequate visualization in a patient with multiple prior surgeries and adhesive disease. In addition, it allows for access to the mid/upper abdomen and the uterine fundus.

   Disadvantages include that it is cosmetically less appealing to the patient, requires increased time to close, and has increased risk of herniation, especially in larger patients. Also as it allows more access to abdominal structures, the bowel may need to be packed to keep it away from the surgical field.[1]

Technique for Midline Vertical Incision

- The skin is incised from below the umbilicus to above the pubic symphysis.
- The subcutaneous fat is then divided until the fascia is encountered.
- A vertical incision is made in the fascia and extended superiorly and inferiorly. Note that this incision will encounter the linea alba and an additional layer of fascia will be excised above this line.
- The peritoneum can then be entered, and the cesarean section proceeds as normal. The closure of the fascia should be with a semipermanent suture such as PDS to allow enough time for the fascia to regain strength. A running mass closure involves all layers of the fascial and muscle wall and allows for a strong, rapid closure.

UTERINE INCISIONS

Lower Uterine Incision and Complications With Anterior Placentation

Transverse incision into the lower uterine segment is the preferred hysterotomy for a cesarean section (Figure 6-7). The obstetrician should review the patient's ultrasound if available to determine the placental position. In a patient with known anterior placentation, the incision should be made below the caudal edge of the placenta. If marginal previa or anterior previa is encountered, the team should be ready for hemorrhage protocol. Techniques for delivery include coming up around the edge of the placenta to deliver the fetus, abrupting and delivering the placenta prior to delivering the fetus,[3] or cutting through the placenta to reach the fetus.[4]

If the placenta is cut through or must be partially separated prior to delivery of the infant, notify the team immediately to prepare for hemorrhage. The obstetrician's focus should be on rapid delivery of the fetus while the team keeps the patient stable.

FUNDAL INCISIONS

A fundal incision may be necessary in cases where the lower uterine segment cannot be exposed or is obstructed due to scar tissue or fibroids. A supraumbilical longitudinal incision may also be the skin incision of choice for morbidly obese and supermorbidly obese patients as discussed in the next section. While this incision allows for access to the uterus without inhibition by the pannus, the surgeon will not be able to reach the lower uterine segment through such a high incision. However, the uterine fundus will be readily available.

In cases where there is extensive scar tissue of the anterior uterus to the abdominal wall, as can sometimes occur with previous cesarean deliveries, the surgeon may choose to do a fundal incision in order to quickly access the fetus or to avoid potential surgical injury such as injury to the bladder. If the anatomy of the uterus is severely distorted by multiple fibroids, a fundal incision may be necessary if this is the only available clear area.

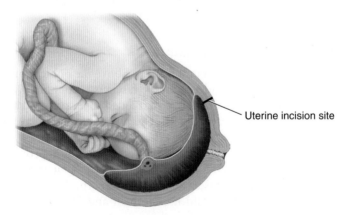

Uterine incision site

FIGURE 6-7 Low transverse hysterotomy with placenta preva. Note that the usual low transverse hysterotomy may be the same level as the placenta in cases of abnormal placentation. (Modified with permission from Stephenson SR. *Obstetrics & Gynecology.* 3rd ed. Philadelphia: Wolters Kluwer; 2013.)

Technique for Fundal Incision

- To perform this incision, the anterior uterine fundus needs to be exposed surgically.
- A scalpel is used to make an incision along the long axis of the anterior uterine fundus (Figure 6-8). The muscle will continue to be cut until the intrauterine cavity is exposed.
- At this point, the incision can either be extended using bandage scissors or carefully continued with the scalpel. The position of the placenta should be known, and the surgeon should keep in mind that anterior fundal is the most likely placental position.
- Similar to delivering around the placenta previa, an attempt should be made to get around the edge of the placenta to reach the fetus. If the placenta must be transverse, be aware that this must be done quickly to decrease maternal and fetal hemorrhage.
- Remember if the baby is in the normal vertex position, this will require a breech delivery. If the fetus is breech, preparation should be made for assistance with a vacuum or forceps as it may be difficult to get traction on the head as an assistant cannot help with pressure to expel the fetus.
- This incision is repaired in the same manner as a classical cesarean section.

Posterior Hysterotomy

Although posterior hysterotomy is exceedingly rare, every obstetrician should have this skill in their arsenal. *The most reported use of the posterior hysterotomy is in the rare case of gestational uterine torsion. This is often an obstetrical emergency and can present with pain and fetal distress.* Uterine torsion can be spontaneous or associated with distortion due to fibroids. Cases have been reported in the literature of torsion up to 180°.

Acute uterine torsion can result in both fetal and maternal distress, and immediate surgical intervention is necessary. An attempt to untorse the uterus can be made, but if this fails, an incision should be made in the lower uterine segment in the transverse or vertical distribution. If the lower uterine segment cannot be accessed, a classical

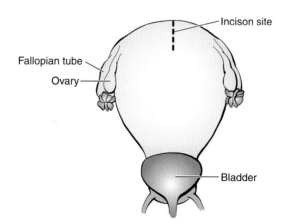

FIGURE 6-8 Fundal incision. The incision extends posteriorly and anteriorly across the top of the uterus. (Modified with permission from Gibbs RS, Karlan BY, Haney AF, Nygaard IE. *Danforth's Obstetrics and Gynecology.* 10th ed. Philadelphia: Wolters Kluwer; 2009.)

cesarean section should be performed to the posterior uterus.[5,6] Other situations in which posterior hysterotomy might be necessary include certain positions of anterior placenta accreta or anterior/fundal uterine fibroids. In these cases, the incision will need to be adequate to allow the uterus to be elevated and expose the posterior portion. A typical classical incision can be made on the exposed portion of the posterior uterus.

SKIN INCISIONS IN THE OBESE PATIENT

It is well documented that obesity continues to rise in the United States.[7] Obesity can create extra difficulties in cesarean section. If a large pannus overlies the suprapubic area, the incision may need to be moved or the pannus elevated to perform the skin incision. Multiple studies have investigated morbidity associated with different incisions, but there is no consensus on what is best for cesarean section. Special precautions for obese patients include assurance that patients are receiving the appropriate dose of antibiotics and considering reapproximation of the subcutaneous fat if measuring more than 2 cm.[8]

Low Transverse Incision

The concern for low transverse incisions in patients who have an overlying pannus include difficulty with access to the area and increased wound infection. The pannus must be elevated and held in place for the procedure to continue. Difficulties may be encountered delivering the fetus as the assistant cannot give adequate fundal pressure because elevation of the pannus increases the adipose tissue above the uterus. Wound infection is always a concern as the area may stay moist, especially if hygiene is an issue.

The advantages of a low transverse incision versus a vertical incision are the patient may have less pain, less risk of herniation, and access for a low transverse hysterotomy to be performed, decreasing the future risk of uterine rupture.

Midline Vertical Incision

This incision is made below the umbilicus to the pubic bone, but the most inferior portion of the pannus is avoided. This incision avoids the problem of having an incision under the pannus. Disadvantages include increased pain and possible increased risk of herniation. In addition, if the subcutaneous tissue is very deep, the lower uterine segment may not be able to be accessed, requiring a fundal or classical uterine incision.

Supraumbilical Transverse Incision

There is a report of good surgical outcomes by performing a transverse incision above the umbilicus in patients whose large pannus displaces the umbilicus inferiorly. The authors report that the lower uterine segment can be easily reached by this report. However, there are not much data on this incision, possibly because of the undesirable cosmetic outcome.[9]

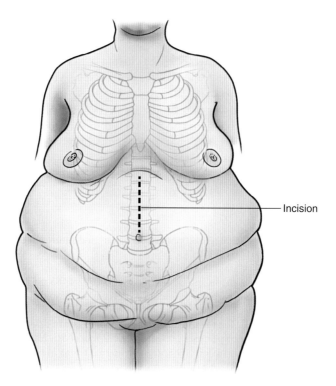

FIGURE 6-9 Supraumbilical longitudinal incision in morbidly obese patient. Note that the umbilicus can be greatly displaced in morbidly obese patients. (Modified with permission from Hatfield NT. *Introductory Maternity and Pediatric Nursing.* 3rd ed. Philadelphia: Wolters Kluwer; 2014.)

Supraumbilical Longitudinal Abdominal Incision

In patients with a body mass index (BMI) over 50 with extreme abdominal adiposity and a large pannus, a supraumbilical longitudinal incision can be considered. In the morbidly obese patient, the supraumbilical region will have the least adipose tissue and therefore be the shortest skin-to-uterus distance (Figure 6-9). Note that this incision usually requires a fundal uterine incision.

PITFALLS

- While separating the fascia from the muscle during a Pfannensteil incision, any perforating vessels encountered should be individually cauterized. If they retract without being properly cauterized, a postoperative rectus hematoma can develop.
- During hysterotomy, if the placenta is cut through or must be partially separated prior to delivery of the infant, notify the team immediately to prepare for hemorrhage.
- The most reported use of the posterior hysterotomy is in the rare case of gestational uterine torsion. This is often an obstetrical emergency and can present with pain and fetal distress.

🛡 **SAFEGUARDS**

- While separating the subcutaneous tissue during a Pfannensteil incision, care must be taken to avoid the superficial epigastric vessels, which run in the subcutaneous tissue just lateral to the rectus muscles.
- The Joel-Cohen low transverse technique can be useful in performing stat cesarean sections as the abdomen can be entered in seconds by an experienced obstetrician. There is a decreased chance of accidentally severing the superficial epigastric vessels and rectus perforating vessels.

REFERENCES

1. Raghavan R, Arya P, Arya P, China S. Abdominal incisions and sutures in obstetrics and gynaecology. *Obstet Gynecol.* 2014;16:13-18.
2. Mathai M, Hofmeyr GJ, Mathai NE. Abdominal surgical incisions for caesarean section. *Cochrane Database Syst Rev.* 2013;(5):CD004453. doi:10.1002/14651858.CD004453.pub3.
3. Ward CR. Avoiding an incision through the anterior previa at cesarean delivery. *Obstet Gynecol.* 2003;102:552-554.
4. Hong DH, Kim E, Kyeon KS, Hong SH, Jeong EH. Safety of cesarean delivery through placental incision in patients with anterior placenta previa. *Obstet Gynecol Sci.* 2016;59(2):103-109.
5. Kim SK, Chung JE, Bai SW, et al. Torsion of the pregnant uterus. *Yonsei Med J.* 2001;42(2):267-269.
6. Moores KL, Wood MG, Foon RP. A rare obstetric emergency; acute uterine torsion in a 32-week pregnancy. *BMJ Case Rep.* 2014;2014.
7. Ogde CL, Carroll MD, Kit BK, Flegal KM. Prevalence of childhood and adult obesity in the United States, 2011-2012. *JAMA.* 2014;311:806-814.
8. Obesity in Pregnancy. Practice bulletin no 156. *Obstet Gynecol.* 2015;126(6):e112-e126. American College of Obstetrics and Gynecologists.
9. Tixier H, Thouvenot S, Coulange L, et al. Cesarean section in morbidly obese women: supra or subumbilica transverse incision? *Acta Obstet Gynecol Scand.* 2009;88:1049-1052.

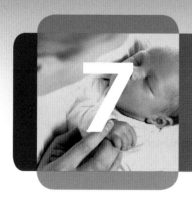

7 Intraoperative Management of Accreta, Percreta, and Increta

Kristy K. Ward

INTRODUCTION

Placenta accreta spectrum (including accreta, increta, and percreta) is one of the most dangerous diagnoses of pregnancy. The depth of chorionic villi invasion characterizes the severity of the placental abnormality, accrete denotes no chorionic invasion, increta is partially invading, and percreta is full-thickness invasion of the myometrium beyond the serosa. In placenta percreta, the abnormal placenta may adhere to the surrounding abdominopelvic organs and musculature. The most common site of attachment is the bladder, but attachment can occur to the rectum and occasionally to the bowel, although this is rare.

After delivery, when the abnormal placenta does not separate from the uterus, postpartum hemorrhage may occur, potentially leading to hemorrhagic shock, coagulopathy, hysterectomy, and death. Average blood loss is between 3000 and 5000 mL and can be much more. Approximately 90% of these patients need a transfusion. Ideally, the delivery of a patient with placenta accreta should be planned and controlled,[1,2] but every obstetrician must be prepared if an unexpected patient with placenta accreta comes into triage.

While placenta accreta spectrum can be one of the most life-threatening pregnancy complications, being prepared with a multidisciplinary plan in place can improve outcomes and decrease provider anxiety. All members of the team should be included in planning and all staff should be aware of protocols. Planning will not only improve management of scheduled deliveries of patients with placenta accreta spectrum, but will also improve management of unexpected deliveries.

THE MULTIDISCIPLINARY TEAM AND PATIENT CONFERENCE

As soon as a patient is identified as having placenta accreta, a multidisciplinary patient conference should be scheduled to formulate a delivery plan. Ideally, members of the team should include the primary obstetrician, a maternal fetal medicine specialist (if not acting as the primary obstetrician), the obstetrical nursing team, obstetrical anesthesia team, a gynecologic oncologist, interventional radiology team, the pediatric/neonatal intensive care unit (NICU) team, the blood bank, the cell saver team, the laboratory, and the ICU team. Urology, trauma/general surgery, and vascular surgery should be aware and available. A contact person should be identified for each of the services. If the hospital has an *accreta team*, the team should be notified.[1,2]

The following include descriptions of the role of each member of the multidisciplinary team.

Primary obstetrician: The primary obstetrician is the head of the team, is primarily responsible for the patient, and leads the patient conference. The obstetrician schedules the cesarean hysterectomy and assures that all members of the team are in place.

Maternal fetal medicine specialist: This specialist diagnoses the placenta accreta and documents location and any possible involved structures. The maternal fetal medicine specialist decides the optimal delivery time and guides the obstetrician in timing of steroids or other interventions.

Obstetrical nursing team: The charge nurse or designated head of the nursing team is responsible for notifying all team members of the delivery and assuring all equipment is available. The nursing team assists in obtaining supplies including blood and labs. One nurse will be responsible for inflating the balloon catheters, if needed.

Gynecologic oncologist: If the primary obstetrician is not experienced in performing high blood loss cesarean hysterectomies, a gynecologic oncologist should be present and responsible for taking charge of the hysterectomy after delivery of the fetus.

Interventional radiology team: The interventional radiology team can place balloon catheters prior to the planned procedure. If it is decided not to use the balloon catheters, the interventional radiologist should be available for embolization of continued bleeding.

Pediatric/NICU team: The NICU team is responsible for the fetus after delivery and is responsible for assuring that all equipment is available, especially if the delivery is performed out of the usual obstetric operating room.

Blood bank: The blood bank should be alerted and prepared for the massive transfusion protocol to be activated.

Cell saver team: If the cell saver is to be used, they will remind the surgeons that all amniotic fluid needs to be cleared prior to using the cell saver. They will operate the machine.

Laboratory: The laboratory should be prepared to run stat samples as needed.

ICU team: A bed needs to be arranged and the ICU team should be expecting to receive the patient after surgery.

Other Team Members to Be Alerted and On-call

The following teams should be aware and on-call for assistance if required:

Urology: The urologist should be available in the case of ureteral or severe bladder injury. If increta involving the urinary tract is known or suspected, the urologist should be involved.

Trauma/General surgery: Additional surgical teams may need to be called depending on the intraoperative findings.

Vascular surgery: The vessels of the pelvis will be engorged and vascular injury is possible. If a vascular injury is encountered, the vascular surgeons should be called as soon as possible (Figure 7-1).

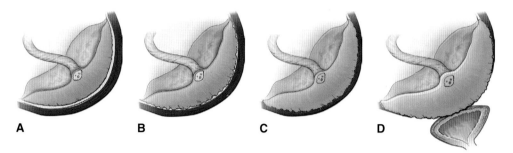

FIGURE 7-1 Placenta accreta spectrum. A, shows normal placental implantation with a normal basal layer. B, shows placenta accreta—there is loss between the placental and maternal interface but no invasion into the myometrium. C, shows placenta increta—the placenta invades into the myometrium but not to the uterine serosa. D, shows placenta percreta—the placenta invades all the way through the myometrium and serosa. In severe cases, the placenta can invade the surrounding tissue such as the bladder.

PLACENTA ACCRETA PLANNED DELIVERY

Preoperative Plan

- The plan should include a preferred delivery age with a scheduled date of delivery (Figure 7-2).
- The patient's hemoglobin should be optimized during the prenatal period.
- A written plan should be formed and placed in a centralized location on labor and delivery.
- A signed hysterectomy consent should be kept with the preoperative plan.
- The admission and delivery date should be planned and scheduled with all teams.
- Appropriate counseling on the morbidity and mortality of placenta accreta should be documented in the prenatal chart.
- Preoperatively, either prior to admission or upon admission to labor and delivery, the patient should meet the gynecologic oncologist, the obstetric anesthesia physician, interventional radiology, and the pediatric/NICU team.[1-3]

Upon Admission

- Upon admission, the patient should receive laboratory work including hemoglobin and hematocrit, creatinine, and a blood type and cross.
- Adequate IV access should be obtained with at least two large bore IVs.
- Appropriate fetal well-being assessments should be performed.

Intraoperative Management[1-3]

- If balloon catheters are to be used, they should be placed just prior to planned surgery.
- The entire team should be present in the room prior to anesthesia induction.
- The patient is prepped and draped and general anesthesia performed.
- A vertical midline incision is created. The uterine incision should be away from the site of the accreta. This will likely require a classical or fundal incision.

CESARIAN HYSTERECTOMY PLAN FOR : (PATIENT NAME)			
MRN:			
EDD:			
Pre op dx:	Accreta	Increta	Percreta
Date/value h/h:			
Date/ value creatinine:			
Date of planned surgery:			
Placenta location:			
Relevant US findings:			
Relevant MRI findings:			
OB history:			
# of previous CD			
pertinent last operative report findings			
other prior uterine surgery			
GA at planned delivery:			
Antenatal steroids given?			
DELIVERY TEAM CONTACT INFORMATION			
	Name	Phone #	Pager/2nd#
OB attending			
OBanesthesia			
MFM attending			
Gyn Onc attending			
Interventional radiology			
Peds/NICU			
Blood bank			
Cell saver			
Lab			
ICU			
Specialty surgical teams:			
Urology			
Trauma/Gen Surg			
Vascular Surg			

FIGURE 7-2 Sample delivery plan template. The template can and should be modified to meet the needs of each specific location and patient.

- After delivery of the fetus, the cord should be clamped with a disposable clamp and placed back in the uterus.
- The uterus should be quickly closed in one layer and the procedure turned over to the gynecologic oncologist (or designated surgeon).
- Do not attempt to remove the placenta in the case of a known accreta/increta/percreta. This can cause life-threatening hemorrhage.
- Surgeon makes the decision of which hysterectomy method. Techniques such as ligating the hypogastric arteries or using the balloon catheters can aid in decreasing blood loss.
- The procedure should be completed as quickly and safely as possible, as blood loss will continue until the uterus is removed.

Unplanned Delivery of Placenta Accreta with a Delivery Plan in Place

One of the greatest advantages of the multidisciplinary conference and delivery plan is the ability to implement it quickly in the case of an emergent delivery. While there is not time to place the balloon catheters, interventional radiology team should still be notified in case their assistance is needed. All members of the team should be called and the delivery should proceed as close to plan as possible.

Unplanned Delivery of an Unknown Placenta Accreta

When an unknown patient comes into triage with bleeding and accreta is discovered during surgery, it can be one of the most dangerous situations encountered in obstetrics. Every labor and delivery should have a plan in place for unknown/emergency placenta accreta.[1-4]

ACCRETA PROTOCOL

- Notify the anesthesiologist of the placenta accreta diagnosis. Make sure it is understood that massive blood loss is eminent and need to call for assistance, get extra lines, and convert to general anesthesia if the patient is awake.
- Notify the circulating nurse to activate the accreta protocol.
- Call the blood bank. Ask the anesthesiologist if the massive transfusion protocol needs to be activated.
- Call the gynecology oncologist or surgeon on call.
- Call the ICU to expect the patient.
- Prepare for hysterectomy. If the hospital does not have the resources to care for the patient, prepare to initiate transfer for higher level of care.
- After the cord is clamped and the uterus is closed, evaluate bleeding. If the bleeding is minimal, close the abdomen and prepare for transfer. If intra-abdominal bleeding can be controlled with packing, the patient may be packed and transferred with the abdomen open. If this fails, hysterectomy must be performed.
- *While the patient and the infant are the team's priority, do not forget that the patient's family is terrified and does not understand what is happening. The family should be given updates as soon as a member of the team is available to do so.*

PLACENTA PERCRETA

Placenta percreta involves the entire myometrium and may penetrate the surrounding organs. These patients often have increased abnormal vasculature on the surface of the uterus. These vessels are very fragile and can quickly contribute to massive blood loss. Holding pressure over the bleeding vessels while performing the hysterectomy can decrease blood loss. In the case of known bladder involvement, a urologist should be involved prenatally to create a plan for removal that likely will involve bladder resection and repair. For bowel involvement, a gynecologic oncologist with experience with bowel repair or a surgeon should be involved. And if the side wall is involved, vascular surgery and interventional radiology will be needed (Figure 7-3).

DELAYED HYSTERECTOMY/FERTILITY SPARING SURGERY

Some institutions have a protocol that involves clamping the cord and closing the uterus with the plan to leave the uterus in place. Delayed hysterectomy can then be performed with the hope for less blood loss. There are also protocols that involve giving methotrexate to allow the placenta to reabsorb in the hopes of preserving fertility. A few case reports discuss segmental excision with over sewing of abnormally adherent placentas. With these options, the majority of patients will need to undergo hysterectomy urgently due to bleeding or infection. Efficacy of these methods is not established and should only be performed in institutions with experience in this setting. *For the majority of obstetricians, leaving the uterus in place should only be considered in cases where transfer to a higher level of care is expected.*[5,6]

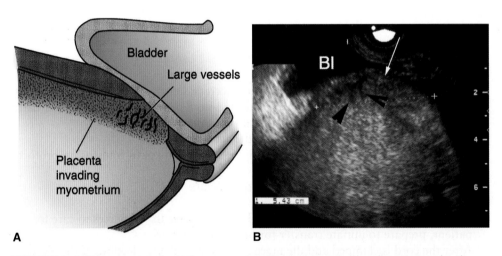

A   **B**

FIGURE 7-3 A, Placenta percreta. At the cesarean section incision site, the placenta invades the myometrium and bladder wall. Large vertically aligned vessels can be seen within the placental invasion site. They may extend into the bladder. B, Placenta percreta; transvaginal view. The placenta previa is entering the myometrium adjacent to the bladder. Note the small, vertically aligned vessels at the percreta site (black arrowheads), which do not run parallel with the myometrium (as in a normal placenta). The myometrium is thin. (Reprinted with permission from Sanders RC. *Clinical Sonography: A Practical Guide.* 5th ed. Wolters Kluwer Health and Pharma; 2015 [Figure 24-24].)

STRATEGIES TO CONTROL BLOOD LOSS

Many of the techniques discussed to decrease blood loss have questionable efficacy in cases of placenta accreta.

Tranexamic Acid

Tranexamic acid prevents fibrin degradation. It has been shown to potentially reduce blood loss in cases of postpartum hemorrhage. It can be given prophylactically after cord clamping, but this has not been proven effective in randomized controlled trials. The recommended dose should not be exceeded as renal cortical necrosis can occur.

Balloon Catheters

Balloon catheters can be placed by interventional radiology into the pelvic vessels. They are left deflated until bleeding occurs, at which time they can be filled. Data is mixed on whether balloon catheters actually prevent blood loss during hysterectomy. They are time consuming and can induce blood clotting of the vessels in rare instances (Figure 7-4).

Uterine Artery Ligation

Uterine artery ligation can be performed quickly and easily in most cases. Care should be taken as the ureter can be very close to the area of ligation. While bilateral uterine artery ligation may decrease uterine bleeding, it will not decrease pelvic bleeding (Figure 7-5).

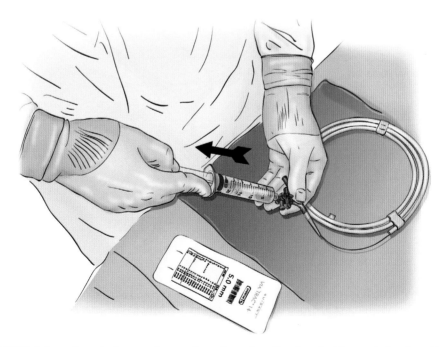

FIGURE 7-4 Prepping a balloon catheter prior to insertion. (Reprinted with permission from Morris PP. *Practical Neuroangiography.* Philadelphia: Wolters Kluwer; 2014.)

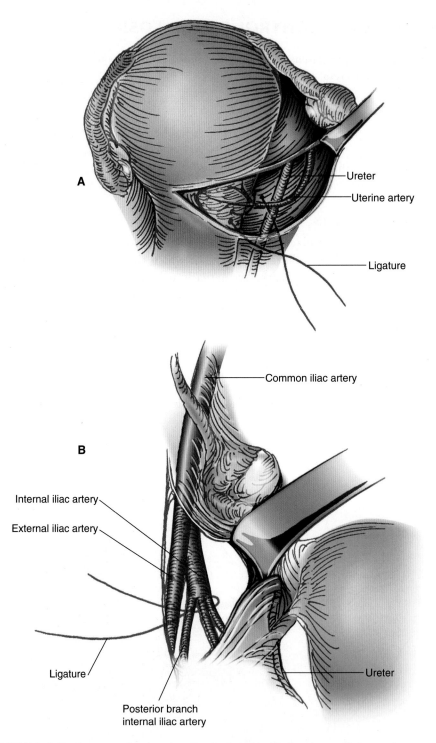

FIGURE 7-5 A, Uterine artery ligation. A suture is placed behind and around the uterine artery lateral to the hysterotomy. B, Hypogastric artery ligation. The hypogastric artery is ligated after branching off of the common iliac. (Reprinted with adaptation from Beckmann CRB. Ling FW, Laube DW, et al. *Obstetrics and Gynecology*. 4th ed. © Wolters Kluwer/LWW; 2002 [Figure 12-2A, B].)

Hypogastric Artery Ligation

Hypogastric artery ligation is used often to control bleeding in pelvic surgery, including cesarean hysterectomy (Figure 7-5B). However, given the large collateral circulation encountered in accreta patients, it may not significantly decrease bleeding in these cases. An experienced pelvic surgeon can usually perform a hypogastric artery ligation quickly, but it can be time consuming and difficult for a surgeon not accustomed to performing this procedure.

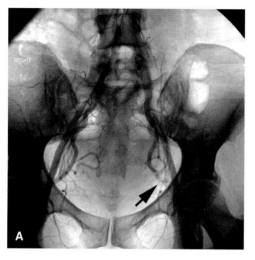
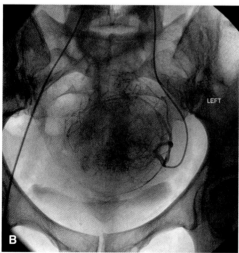
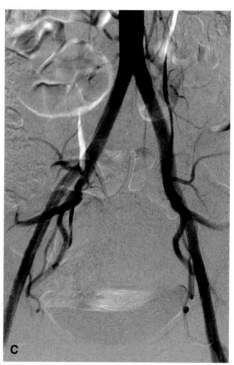

FIGURE 7-6 Uterine artery embolization. A, Pelvic angiogram shows bleeding from a uterine vessel on the left (arrow). B, Embolic particles are selectively injected into the uterine arteries. C, Post-embolization angiogram shows the bleeding to have been stopped. Compare with A. (Reprinted with permission from Daffner RH, Hartman M. *Clinical Radiology*. 4th ed. Wolters Kluwer Health and Pharma/LWW; 2013 [Figure 3.30A-C].)

Postoperative Vessel Embolization Performed by Interventional Radiology

While this is an effective strategy for controlling postoperative bleeding, the patient must be stable enough to undergo the procedure (Figure 7-6A to C). Unfortunately, the majority of accreta patients will not be stable enough to consider this option.

Abdominal Packing

In cases where bleeding cannot be controlled surgically, especially when disseminated intravascular coagulation is encountered, it may be necessary to place intra-abdominal packing, leave the abdomen open, and monitor the patient in the ICU until her hematologic status improves. There are many techniques for packing the abdomen, including using gauze, sterile bags, and specialized vacuum devices (Figure 7-7). Packing is left in place for 24 to 48 hours and then the patient returns to the operating room for removal and closure (Figure 7-7). This may allow the patient to be stabilized enough to consider interventional radiological embolization.[1-3]

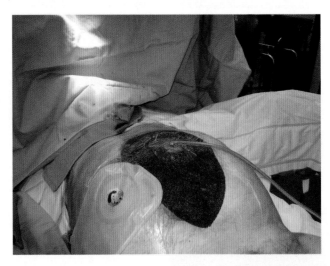

FIGURE 7-7 Abdominal packing. The abdomen is packed with surgical gauze and a dressing placed to hold the gauze. In this example, vacuum tubing is seen at the top of the dressing to help drain the accumulation of fluid. (From Britt. *Acute Care Surgery*. Wolters Kluwer; 2019.)

 PITFALLS

- Do not attempt to remove the placenta in the case of a known accreta/increta/percreta. This can cause life-threatening hemorrhage.
- Many of the techniques discussed to decrease blood loss have questionable efficacy in cases of placenta accreta.

🛡 SAFEGUARDS

- When an unknown patient comes into triage with bleeding and accreta is discovered during surgery, it can be one of the most dangerous situations encountered in obstetrics. Every labor and delivery should have a plan in place for unknown/emergency placenta accreta.
- While the patient and the infant are the team's priority, do not forget that the patient's family is terrified and does not understand what is happening. The family should be given updates as soon as a member of the team is available to do so.
- For the majority of obstetricians, leaving the uterus in place should only be considered in cases where transfer to a higher level of care is expected.[5,6]

REFERENCES

1. Placenta Accreta Spectrum. Obstetric Care Consensus. American College of Obstetrics and Gynecologists and Society for Maternal-Fetal Medicine. *Obstet Gynecol.* 2018;132(6):e259-e275.
2. Shamshirsaz A, Salmanian B, Fox K, et al. Maternal morbidity in patient with morbidly adherent placenta treated with and without a multidisciplinary approach. *Am J Obstet Gynecol.* 2014;1:e1-e19.
3. Silver R, Fox K, Barton J, et al. Center for excellence for placenta accreta. *Am J Obstet Gynecol.* 2015;212(5):561-568. doi:10.1016/j.ajog.2014.11.018.
4. Bowman Z, Manuck T, Eller A, Simons M, Silver R. Risk factors for unscheduled delivery in patients with placenta accreta. *Am J Obstet Gynecol.* 2014;241:e1-e6.
5. Fox KA, Shamshiraz AA, Carusi D, et al. Conservative management of morbidly adherent placenta: expert review. *Am J Obstet Gynecol.* 2015;213:755-760.
6. Perez-Delboy A, Wright JD. Surgical management of plancenta accrete: to leave or remove the placenta? *Br J Obstet Gynecol.* 2014;121:163-169.

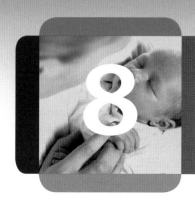

8 Peripartum Hysterectomy

Todd Boren, Sarah Boyd, Stephen DePasquale, C. David Adair

INTRODUCTION AND HISTORICAL PERSPECTIVE

Puerperal, obstetric, or peripartal hysterectomy implies the surgical removal of the uterus of a patient that is either currently or recently pregnant. The technique was advanced in the late 19th century as means to address infection, hemorrhage, and facilitation of indicated cesarean delivery, all of which carried an almost uniform outcome of maternal death. Earlier, the surgical removal of the problematic uterus was the only way to save a mother. With the advent of modern antisepsis, anesthesia, blood transfusion capability, and antibiotics, both hysterectomy and subsequently an evolution to true cesarean delivery became a reality. Since the advent of the newfound safe cesarean delivery, the need for hysterectomy was largely relegated to a lifesaving intervention for treatment of hemorrhagic complications.

With an improved surgical armamentarium and safe cesarean delivery, obstetric hysterectomy significantly decreased in its utilization during most of the 20th century. This was due largely to an increase in cesarean delivery being accomplished with the retention of the recently gravid uterus with excellent safety and ease. The timeliness of this chapter serves us well to reflect upon the recent increased rate of obstetric hysterectomy. The increased rate may largely be associated with the morbidly adherent placenta which occurs mainly from prior cesarean delivery. While the obstetrician is well versed on the technique of hysterectomy, the obstetric hysterectomy requires special attention to anatomical distortion due to pregnancy or its complications such as uterine rupture and tears, blood volume and flow aberrations commonly associated with hemorrhage secondary to either uterine atony or morbid adherence of the placenta. This is particularly of concern with the US cesarean section rates approaching one in three births and increasing likelihood of repeat cesarean once the first one has been performed. These procedures lead to significant increased risks of hemorrhagic complications and morbid adherence of the placenta. The surgical approach and management of these cases require special preparation, technique, and both intra- and post-op care provision.

Planned Versus Unplanned Peripartum Hysterectomy

The peripartum hysterectomy can be challenging. To ensure optimal patient outcomes, our opinion is that planned or anticipated procedures should be scheduled in centers accustomed to level one trauma, generally consistent with a maternal level of care 3 or 4.[1] A multidisciplinary operative team, with adequate intensive care support for postoperative management is critical. Ideally, these patients, if diagnosed with abnormal placentation prior to delivery, are transferred to the appropriate higher-level care center. Preoperative surgical planning includes the assembly of the proper team and availability of multiple units and types of blood products with a massive transfusion protocol in place.

If the need for cesarean hysterectomy is unexpectedly required, one of the most urgent portions of the procedure is to make the decision to proceed to hysterectomy prior to development of a consumptive coagulopathy. Once the decision and hysterectomy are required, efficiently expediting the procedure will minimize blood loss and improve patient outcomes.

PREOPERATIVE SURGICAL PLANNING

Indications for peripartum hysterectomy include uterine hemorrhage, abnormal placentation, infection, uterine anomalies, uterine rupture, and rarely malignancy. The procedure may be anticipated and planned accordingly as an indicated elective procedure or it may be emergent in nature, thus largely unplanned.

The most common indication for a planned peripartum hysterectomy is the spectrum of abnormal placentation; previa, placenta accreta, increta, or percreta (see Chapter 4, **Abnormal Placentation after Cesarean Delivery**). Approximately 60% of patients with abnormal placentation will require a hysterectomy at time of delivery.[2] The incidence of placenta accreta has increased significantly over the past several decades with the main risk factors including prior cesarean section and placental previa.[3]

The most common indication for an emergent peripartum hysterectomy is severe uterine hemorrhage due to uterine atony or abnormal placentation the latter of which accounts for 30% to 50% of peripartum hysterectomies[3-7] (Figure 8-1). Less frequently, a pelvic abscess following cesarean delivery can result in a peripartum hysterectomy

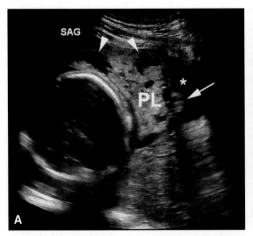
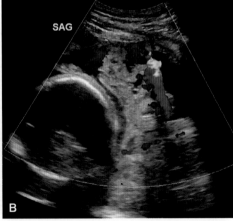

FIGURE 8-1 Ultrasound demonstration of morbidly adherent placentation. Arrowheads indicate sonolucencies seen in PAS; arrow indicates placenta bulging into bladder; and asterisk indicates bladder. (From Doubilet PM, Benson CB, Benacerraf BR. Wolters Kluwer Health and Pharma. 2018.)

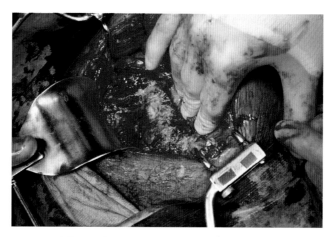

FIGURE 8-2 Postcesarean delivery abscess. (From Sweet RL, Gibbs RS. *Atlas of Infectious Diseases of the Female Genital Tract*. Philadelphia: Lippincott Williams & Wilkins; 2005.)

(Figure 8-2). The peripartum hysterectomy differs from a hysterectomy done for gynecologic indications in several ways. In pregnancy, the uterus receives approximately 20% of the cardiac output resulting in dilated and tortuous blood vessels as well as varices in the vesicouterine space and mesosalpinx. Disruption of these friable vessels can result in significant hemorrhage and a compromised operative field. The peripartum cervix is often soft and difficult to palpate accurately. This may result in unintended retention of portions of cervical or endometrial tissue. Tissue integrity in the pelvis is commonly compromised due to edema and inflammation resulting in shearing of clamped blood vessels. Cognizance of these pregnancy-induced influences and anticipation of managing potential complications can lead to improved outcomes.

Facility and Team

Ideally, the location where a peripartum hysterectomy takes place should be such that all necessary resources are present and easily accessible. Typically, a level 3 or level 4 maternal facility are where these resources are readily available and include adequately trained anesthesia staff capable of medically managing massive hemorrhage, intensive care services, adequate blood product availability, and appropriate ancillary staff such as experienced surgical technicians and nurse circulators paired with a dedicated team of consultative services, such as maternal fetal medicine, gynecologic oncology, urology, trauma surgery, vascular surgery, and interventional radiology. A separate dedicated team should be available to manage blood product transfusion in the appropriate proportions with activation of a massive blood transfusion protocol when needed. A massive blood transfusion protocol with a separate member of the team will ensure correct and accurate ratio of blood product replacement. Every attempt should be made preoperatively to attain adequate intravenous access. Significant fluid shifts often occur during a peripartum hysterectomy in the form of crystalloid and blood product infusion as well as intra- and postoperative blood loss and third spacing. Therefore, adequate hemodynamic monitoring is critical, and as such, if a peripartum hysterectomy is planned, placement of an arterial line and a central line prior to starting the procedure is essential. When a peripartum hysterectomy becomes a necessity as a result of unexpected hemorrhage, then central venous access should be attained as quickly as possible; hence the need for experienced and qualified anesthesia personnel.

Operative Suite and Equipment

Preoperative planning for a peripartum hysterectomy should ensure appropriate and adequate equipment availability to manage every possible outcome that may occur. Adequate preoperative preparation is just as important as intraoperative skill and judgment and every effort should be made to have the entire team assembled and available prior to incision.

- Surgical illumination of the operative suite is critical and should be fully equipped with proper overhead lighting.
- Surgeon mounted headlamps aid greatly in proper visualization of pelvic structures and are particularly useful when significant bleeding is encountered.
- Authors use a self-retaining retractor, such as the Bookwalter retractor, which facilitates adequate visualization.
- Electrocautery and a vessel-sealing device such as a LigaSure Impact Open Sealer/Divider (Medtronic, Boulder, Colorado) should be available (Figure 8-3).
- Authors find that the utilization of Zeppelin clamps during the hysterectomy minimizes the potential for tissue or blood vessel slippage.
- Equipment for urological evaluation and management should be readily available to facilitate stent placement or evaluate for suspected urinary tract injury including a cystoscope, ureteral stents, and fluoroscopy.
- Interventional radiology suite may prove to be invaluable for preoperative placement of vascular catheters or postoperative embolization.
- Hemostatic agents can be very useful in the setting of peripartum hemorrhage or disseminated intravascular coagulopathy. Evesil and Arista secondary to their effectiveness and ease of application or similar products should be made immediately available. These agents have proven to be of great assistance in our collective experience.
- Suture offerings of various size and material should be available. We prefer to utilize either Monocrylor Vicryl sutures. Both offer excellent tensile strength and provide the surgeon with minimal tissue shearing.
- Large bore drains may be considered, as it may inform the postoperative care team early warning of bleeding persistence or recurrence. A 19 French round Blake drain(s) usually proves more than adequate.

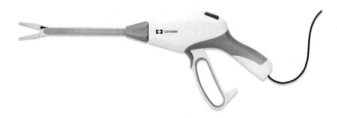

FIGURE 8-3 LigaSure Impact Open Sealer/Divider. (© Medtronic, Boulder, Colorado)

CHOICE OF SKIN INCISION IN PERIPARTUM HYSTERECTOMY

When the indication for peripartum hysterectomy arises and a Pfannenstiel incision has been made, our approach is to extend the incision by either dividing the rectus muscles (Maylard incision) or performing a Cherney incision as outlined below. Conversion of a Pfannenstiel incision to either a Maylard or Cherney incision should provide more than adequate exposure to perform all aspects of a peripartum hysterectomy. We feel it is imperative to emphasize this, as inadequate exposure can result in injury to pelvic structures and delayed hemostasis.

Procedure for Converting from Pfannenstiel Incision to a Maylard Incision:

- With the Maylard approach, an Army-Navy retractor can be placed underneath the rectus muscle between the posterior aspect of the muscle and the peritoneum.
- Using electrocautery, the muscle is then divided. The inferior epigastric artery becomes more lateral in the rectus muscle as you approach the pubic symphysis. Identification of this artery is paramount, and it is either ligated with a suture ligature or a vessel sealer prior to transection.
- Note of caution: if the inferior epigastric artery is inadvertently lacerated, it can retract into the muscle making it very recalcitrant and very difficult to control bleeding.
- Closure of the Maylard incision is accomplished by reapproximating the inferior and superior ends of the rectus muscle belly with two 2-0 PDS sutures on each side placed in a horizontal mattress fashion.
- Closure of the peritoneum may decrease the risk of the bowel attaching to exposed muscle as well in this particular situation.
- The fascia can then be closed over the top of the reapproximated muscle ends with #1 PDS suture in a running fashion.

Procedure for Converting from a Pfannenstiel Incision to a Cherney Incision:

- The lateral margins of the skin incision should extend out several centimeters. The insertions of the rectus muscle tendons to the pubic symphysis should be identified.
- The rectus muscle tendons are then transected at their midpoint with electrocautery. Just lateral to the rectus muscle tendon, the inferior epigastric artery emerges from the lateral aspect of the rectus muscle.
- Prior to mobilizing the rectus muscles superiorly, the inferior epigastric arteries must be either ligated with suture and divided or alternatively transected with a commercially available vessel-sealing device.
- The rectus muscles can then be mobilized superiorly and a generous peritoneal incision can be made.
- Following closure of a Cherney incision, one should reattach the inferior and superior ends of the rectus tendons with two horizontal mattress sutures on each tendon using a 2-0 PDS suture.

CHOICE OF UTERINE INCISION

During a cesarean section, a transverse uterine incision is typically performed to decrease the risk of uterine rupture in subsequent pregnancies and to allow for the possibility of future vaginal deliveries. In general, the authors prefer a uterine vertical incision in cases where a peripartum hysterectomy is anticipated. In cases of known abnormal placentation, the authors prefer a fundal incision, starting at the superior aspect of the uterus and carrying the incision over the fundus and ending on the posterior aspect of the uterus with delivery of the fetus through the open fundus. This technique often avoids disruption of the pathologically adherent placenta during fetal delivery and in turn minimizes blood loss prior to the hysterectomy portion of the procedure. If hysterectomy is planned or likely secondary to abnormal placentation, prior knowledge of placentation is critical. Equally important is to not disrupt the placenta, in an effort aimed at attempting to minimize blood loss. Customization of the uterine incision is based on a preoperative ultrasound to confirm location of the placenta, again in an attempt to minimize potential for placenta disruption.

A recent report by Belfort et al., describes a technique using a GIA stapler to make the hysterotomy.[8]

New Technique Using a GIA Stapler to Make the Hysterotomy (Figures 8-4 and 8-5)

- Four sutures are placed at right angles to each other through the myometrium creating an avascular window through which electrocautery is used to dissect down to the amniotic sac.
- The plane between the amniotic sac and myometrium is bluntly dissected in the direction of the intended hysterotomy incision, and one arm of the GIA stapler is guided along this plane.
- The other arm of the stapler is connected, and once fired, a double layer of staples is laid down and a retractable blade makes a myometrial incision between the staple lines. This creates a hemostatic hysterotomy incision through which the fetus can be delivered with significantly less blood loss as compared to a traditional hysterotomy incision.
- Then the incision can be closed in the usual fashion with a running stitch or alternatively several figure-of-8 sutures just prior to proceeding with the hysterectomy.

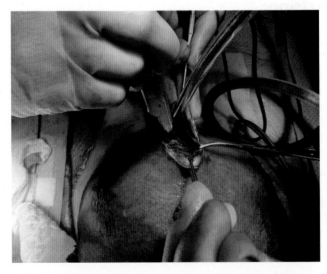

FIGURE 8-4 Initial hysterotomy opening in anticipation of GIA Stapler.

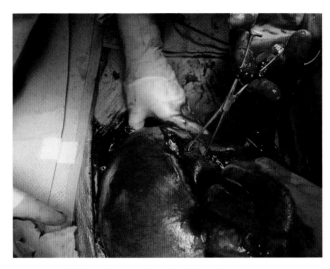

FIGURE 8-5 GIA Stapler completed and amniotomy commencement.

Authors' Modification

The authors recently have made a slight modification to this technique. Prior to making the small hysterotomy incision to dissect down the amniotic sac, we perform an ultrasound evaluation of the placental location with the ultrasound probe directly on the myometrial surface. Once the borders of the placenta have been identified, small cautery marks are made on the serosal surface that coincide with the placental border which provides a "map" of the placental location on the serosal surface of the uterus. With this information, the GIA stapler can be oriented in a way that will not disrupt the placenta and minimizes blood loss.

OPERATIVE TECHNIQUES FOR PERIPARTUM HYSTERECTOMY

Traditional Technique for Peripartum Hysterectomy

The traditional technique for performing a peripartum hysterectomy has been described in several publications.[9-11]

- The general description first starts by isolating the round ligament and by making an incision in the anterior and posterior broad ligaments (Figure 8-6).
- The round ligaments are then doubly clamped, transected, and then doubly ligated with suture placement on the lateral aspect.
- Other authors have made special mention that Sampson artery is inconsequential in most gynecologic procedures but can result in significant bleeding if not properly secured and ligated in a peripartum hysterectomy.
- The vascular bundles in the uterine ovarian ligaments are isolated by making a blunt or sharp rent in the posterior broad ligament.
- These vascular bundles are then clamped and transected sharply, and the medial and lateral pedicles are ligated with # 0 or #1 suture material. The lateral pedicles should be doubly ligated secondary to the congested ovarian arteries and veins.
- Alternatively, after a single ligature is placed behind the most lateral clamp on the lateral pedicle, a stitch may be placed in the midportion of the pedicle between the ligature and the remaining clamp.

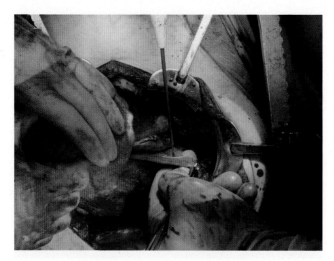

FIGURE 8-6 Round ligament division.

- The ends of the suture can then be brought around the tip of the clamp in opposite directions and then tied behind the clamp thus transfixing the pedicle and preventing slippage of tissue and vessels.
- Traditionally, the fallopian tubes are left attached to the ovaries by the mesosalpinx after being transected at the uterine cornua along with the ovarian vessels (modification to this technique is discussed later).
- Next, the bladder flap is developed except in cases of suspected bladder invasion or involvement.
- The vesicouterine peritoneum is incised by electrocautery lateral to medial starting at the transected edge of the anterior broad ligament.
- The two incisions are connected in the midline and the avascular vesicouterine space is then developed bluntly. Note, however, that sharp dissection may be necessary if adhesions are present from prior cesarean sections. *Care must be taken not to disrupt the venous sinuses that are present laterally in the uterine vesicular pillars as these veins are usually very congested and, given their close proximity to the ureters, bleeding from them can be difficult to safely control.*
- Once the bladder is mobilized and caudad, the uterine artery and vein are identified near the cervical isthmus between the anterior and posterior leaves of the broad ligament.
- A sharply curved or right-angle clamp is then placed across the uterine vessels at a right angle to the vessels, and two additional clamps are placed beneath the original clamp. The ureters can be in close proximity to the placement of these clamps and traction of the uterus in a direction opposite of the side of the vessels being clamped can help displace the vessels away from the ureter passing beneath.
- The vessels are then transected between the most medial clamp and the lateral two clamps, which allows for two suture ligatures to be placed on the lateral pedicle. This placement helps to avoid slippage of the vascular bundle and significant bleeding.
- *In an ideal situation, the surgeon's hand is then placed around the lower uterine segment and the distal end of the cervix is palpated, a process which marks the distal end of the bladder dissection and the limits of the cardinal ligament transection. However, the cervix in a peripartum hysterectomy is often difficult to palpate accurately, especially if it is significantly effaced with prior labor.*

- At this point a *supracervical hysterectomy* can be performed. Placentation again is critical. Supracervical hysterectomy may not be appropriate with placenta previa. The cervix is amputated at a level just beneath the ligated uterine vessels. The cervical stump can then be over sewn in an imbricating fashion using interrupted or continuous sutures.

Complete Hysterectomy: Step-by-step Approach

- The distal end of the cervix must be identified. If the distal cervix cannot be located by palpation, then several methods have been described to accomplish this goal. A vertical midline incision can be made in the lower uterine segment and a finger passed through this incision to identify the vaginal fornices (Figure 8-7). Alternatively, four metal skin clips or brightly colored sutures can be placed at the 12, 3, 6, and 9 o'clock locations on the distal cervix prior to the surgery. Another alternative to technique for locating the vaginal fornices is described under section on Modifications.
- Once the distal cervix of vaginal fornices have been identified, straight Zeppelin clamps are placed across the cardinal ligaments in a vertical fashion as close to the cervix as possible, starting just medial to the lateral pedicle containing the uterine vessels.
- The cardinal ligament is then transected medial to the straight clamp, and the pedicles are then secured with a suture ligature. This process is repeated successively until the level of the cervicovaginal junction is reached.
- The bladder is then reassessed, and care is taken to make sure that the vesicouterine space has been developed caudad to the distal end of the cervix.
- A right-angle clamp is then placed across the lateral vaginal fornix and uterosacral ligament just beneath the level of the cervix while a contralateral clamp is placed in similar fashion. Alternatively, the uterosacral ligaments can be clamped, transected, and secured with a suture ligature separately prior to placing the right-angle clamp.
- The tissue anterior to the clamps is transected and the specimen removed.

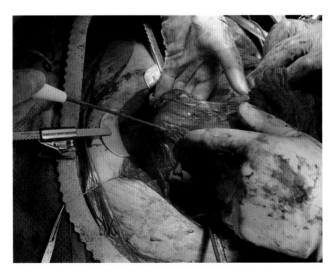

FIGURE 8-7 Palpation of vaginal fornixes.

- The cervix is then examined to ensure it has been completely excised.
- Utilizing a Haney stitch, the left and right pedicles containing the lateral vagina and uterosacral ligaments are secured, if not transected previously.
- The remaining vaginal edges are reapproximated with either interrupted or continuous suture.
- All pedicles are then reexamined for hemostasis. Bleeding at the lateral margins of the vaginal cuff can be controlled with suture ligatures but caution must be taken to avoid the ureter at this location. Of note, we prefer to leave all suture ends to be marginally longer than normal. This allows for pedicle identification in cases necessitating surgical re-exploration to be a useful practice.

MODIFICATIONS TO THE TRADITIONAL TECHNIQUE FOR PERIPARTUM HYSTERECTOMY

Preoperative Ureteral Catheter Placement

The first modification we describe involves routine placement of temporary ureteral catheters prior to starting a planned peripartum hysterectomy. Using a cystoscope, open-ended ureteral catheters are placed through each ureteral orifice and advanced to the renal pelvis (Figure 8-8). Placement of open-ended ureteral catheters helps facilitate digital palpation of the ureter when placing clamps and suture ligatures and can help avoid ureteral injury. The Foley catheter is then replaced, and the open-ended ureteral catheters are attached to the Foley catheter to keep them in place. We recommend visual identification of the ureters intraoperatively; however, due to significant bleeding, patient habitus, or anatomic derangements, visual inspection of ureteral location may not be feasible. If a clamp is accidently placed across the ureter, then the clamp can be removed. The presence of the open-ended ureteral catheter then allows for convenient placement of a double J ureteral stent through the injured ureter. If the ureter is inadvertently transected, the injury is more easily recognizable with a yellow open-ended ureteral catheter in place and the proximal and distal transected ends are more identifiable. Following the hysterectomy, the catheters are easily removed either separately or along with the Foley catheter whenever deemed

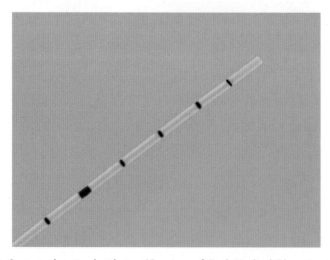

FIGURE 8-8 Open-end ureteral catheter. (Courtesy of Cook Medical, Bloomington, Indiana.)

appropriate. We often leave the open-ended ureteral catheters for the first 24 hours. Once hemostasis is assured, they can easily be removed at the bedside. The open-ended ureteral catheters are usually placed following induction of general anesthesia. Alternatively, they can be placed while the cesarean section is being performed in cases of active bleeding. In a situation where hysterectomy is unplanned secondary to unanticipated abnormal placentation or irretractable bleeding, the catheters can be placed cystoscopically by an assistant while hemostasis is being rendered through the abdominal incision.

Elective or Opportunistic Salpingectomy

Traditional descriptions of peripartum hysterectomy have stated to leave the fallopian tubes attached to the ovaries via the mesosalpinx when the uterine ovarian ligament is transected. There appears to be a moderate decrease in the risk of epithelial ovarian cancer in patients who undergo complete salpingectomy versus traditional sterilization methods.[12] In addition, there does not appear to be an increase in operative complications or a decrease in ovarian reserve associated with complete salpingectomy versus traditional sterilization methods.[13,14] As such, we recommend performing a complete bilateral salpingectomy at the time of peripartum hysterectomy, of course in patients who are hemodynamically stable and in absence of consumptive coagulopathy. This procedure can be accomplished by clamping the vessels in the mesosalpinx and then securing the mesosalpinx pedicle on the ovarian side with 2-0 sutures. Alternatively, the mesosalpinx vessels can be taken with a vessel-sealing device as described below.

Modifications Using Vessel-Sealing Devices

Traditional methods of securing vascular pedicles during a peripartum hysterectomy involve placing metal clamps across the pedicles and then securing the transected pedicles with braided or monofilament sutures. The increased size of peripartum uterine and ovarian vessels and their branches as well as the significant edema present in surrounding tissue can result in slippage of the clamped vascular pedicle or shearing of clamped vessels resulting in significant hemorrhage. In an effort to decrease these risks, we have begun to utilize the use of a vessel-sealing device to secure the majority of vascular pedicles when performing a peripartum hysterectomy. We have found the LigaSure vessel-sealing devices to have ease of use and minimal lateral spread of tissue desiccation (Figure 8-3). There is less than 2 mm of lateral tissue damage produced by the LigaSure device and is comparable to the harmonic scalpel.[15] We have found increased surgical efficiency is particularly useful in cases of significant hemorrhage when pedicles must be secured quickly and effectively.

Technique for Use of a Vessel-Sealing Device to Secure Majority of Vascular Pedicles

- Application of the vessel-sealing device during a peripartum hysterectomy starts with transecting the mesosalpinx when performing a bilateral salpingectomy.
- After the fallopian tubes are removed, the vascular bundle containing the uterine ovarian vessels can then be transected using the vessel sealer device. Most vessel-sealing devices can successfully seal and transect vessels up to 7 mm in diameter or less. Even with the vascular dilation that results from pregnancy, the ovarian artery and vein are typically less than 7 mm in diameter.

- When securing the uterine artery and vein at the cervical isthmus we still prefer to use right angle Zeppelin clamps and suture ligatures as the uterine vessels, the veins in particular, can easily exceed 7 mm in diameter.
- After the uterine vessels are secured, we find that the cardinal ligament can be safely and efficiently taken down to the level of the external cervix by continued use of the vessel-sealing device. The ureter is 2 cm lateral to the cervix at this location and there is minimal risk of thermal damage, however, the ureter should still be either visualized or palpated prior to applying any thermal energy or clamp to the cardinal ligament.

Use of Vessel-Sealing Device With Bladder Placental Invasion

Abnormal placentation with placental invasion into the bladder provides for another very useful application of a vessel-sealing device. When a percreta is suspected, cystoscopy is performed intraoperatively to determine the location of bladder involvement. We do not attempt to develop the vesicouterine space in this situation. Instead, a cystotomy is made in the bladder dome in a location determined by cystoscopic evaluation not to be involved with placental tissue. The trigone and ureteral orifices are easily identified with the Pollack catheters in place. Using the vessel-sealing device, the area of bladder containing ectopic placental tissue is excised with care taken to avoid the bladder trigone and ureteral orifices. We find that this technique dramatically reduces blood loss in cases of placenta percreta.

Video 8-1
Anterior colpotomy on KOH ring.

Use of the Koh Cup Ring to Identify the Vaginal Fornix

As mentioned above, identifying the distal end of the cervix and vaginal fornix can be very challenging during a peripartum hysterectomy secondary to laboring forces and tissue edema. Below we describe a novel and effective method to accurately delineate the vaginal fornices using the KOH Colpotomizer Cups (Cooper Surgical Inc, Trumbull, Connecticut) (Figure 8-9).[16]

- The procedure begins by performing a vaginal examination to access the vaginal capacity and cervical size. Typically, our first choice is the largest KOH Cup that the vagina will accommodate to make palpation of the KOH Cup edges as easy as possible from the abdominal side of the vagina.
- The KOH Cup can be placed into the vagina and around the cervix, at the time of cystoscopy and ureteral catheters placement. The KOH Cup can easily be oriented to allow for accurate and simple palpation of the KOH Cup edges, allowing for easier identification of the pregnant cervix.
- Once the bladder flap has been developed and the cardinal ligaments transected to the appropriate level, the circular edge of the KOH Cup is then identified and a circumferential colpotomy incision is made along the KOH Cup edge using electrocautery (Figure 8-10).
- The uterine specimen is then removed.
- By using this method, the location of the vaginal fornices can be accurately and efficiently identified, which allows for consistent colpotomy placement and in turn minimizes the risk of retained cervical tissue or excessive vaginal tissue removal. The vagina and uterosacral ligaments are then reapproximated as described previously.

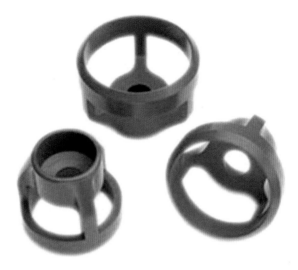

FIGURE 8-9 KOH Colpotomizer Cups. (Cooper Surgical Inc, Trumbull, Connecticut)

MANAGEMENT OF BLADDER AND URETERAL INJURIES

Most patients who present with abnormal placentation have undergone multiple prior cesarean sections. In addition, these patients have increased risk of injury to genitourinary structures and significant adhesive disease in the pelvis, which can cause anatomic distortion for pelvic organs. A recent meta-analysis reported a 10% risk of genitourinary complications including bladder or ureteral injury and fistula formation among 5704 women who underwent peripartum hysterectomy.[17] Kwee et al. reported an 8% risk of bladder injury in patients undergoing peripartum hysterectomy.[18]

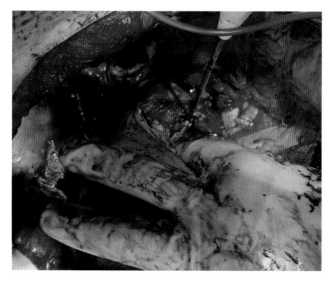

FIGURE 8-10 Electrocautery entry on the KOH ring cup of the cervix.

The most important aspect of managing a genitourinary injury is accurately identifying the injury itself; therefore, every effort should be made to continuously evaluate the bladder and ureters during a peripartum hysterectomy to minimize the risk of injury and to maximize to chances of identifying an injury should one occur. (See additional information in Chapter 9: Urologic and Gastrointestinal Injuries.) In the event of a suspected bladder injury, the bladder is filled with normal saline or sterile infant formula in a retrograde manner through a Foley catheter. Most bladder injuries are easily identified using this method. Alternatively, methylene blue dye can be applied to the normal saline to make any bladder defect more apparent. However, it is important to note that these dyes can lead to tissue discoloration inhibiting future tissue delineation. Once identified, the relationship of the cystotomy to the ureteral orifices can easily be determined with Pollack catheters in place. If the ureters have not been previously catheterized and the cystotomy is suspected to be close to the trigone, one ampule of indigo carmine dye can be given intravenously, and the ureteral orifices can be identified by the efflux of blue urine seen through the cystotomy. If the cystotomy is less than 2 cm away from either ureteral orifice, we recommend placing a double J ureteral stent prior to closure. The stent can then be removed in 4 to 6 weeks. The cystotomy is closed in two layers using 2-0 braided or monofilament suture. The first layer is a full-thickness running stitch through the bladder mucosa starting on both sides of the bladder defect and the ends of the suture are tied in the middle of the defect. The second layer is an imbricating running stitch incorporating the detrusor muscle and bladder serosa done in a similar manner. The bladder is then filled in a retrograde fashion to confirm fluid integrity. A Foley catheter is placed and can be removed in 10 to 14 days after a normal retrograde cystogram.

If a ureteral injury is suspected, the type, location, and extent of the injury should be determined before any repair efforts are undertaken. If a crush injury is suspected by placement of an errant clamp, the clamp should be removed immediately, and the ureter inspected. If the ureter does not appear to be transected, a double J ureteral stent can be placed and then removed in 4 to 6 weeks. Removal and reanastomosis of the clamped ureter is typically not necessary if the clamp is removed promptly. Suspected ureteral transections or luminal injuries can be evaluated in several ways. For example, direct visualization can be accomplished by ureterolysis down to the point of suspected injury. Urine efflux is often seen at the point of injury, and if the injury is not so apparent, indigo carmine can be given intravenously as blue urine may be easier to identify at the site of injury. Additionally, the ureter can be cannulated in a retrograde fashion via a cystoscope and any injury or obstruction of the ureter can be identified.

Although a detailed description of repair procedures on the ureter is beyond the scope of this chapter, several points should be made.

1. Ueteral injuries that occur within 5 cm of the bladder can be repaired with an ureteroneocystostomy using a psoas hitch or a Boari flap. See Figures 9.5 and 9.6 in Chapter 9: Urologic and Gastrointestinal Injuries.
2. Ureteral injuries greater than 5 cm from the bladder are usually repaired using a ureteroureterostomy. See end-to-end ureteroureterostomy in Figure 9.7.

3. In both cases, the repair must be tension free and hemostatic, while the anastomotic portion of the ureter must have a wide enough aperture to minimize the risk of stricture.

4. All repairs are performed over a double J ureteral stent, which is left in place for 4 to 6 weeks.

MANAGEMENT OF INTRAOPERATIVE BOWEL INJURIES

Fortunately, bowel injuries are a rare event during peripartum hysterectomies, occurring in less than 3% of cases.[13] However, unidentified bowel injuries can have catastrophic consequences thus appropriate evaluation of the GI tract should be performed throughout the procedure and any injuries promptly identified should then occur. Once identified, the location, size, and extent of the injury should be determined. Minor serosal defects on the surface of the large or small intestine can be closed with either interrupted or a running 2-0 silk suture in a single layer. Full-thickness injuries to the small bowel can typically be closed primarily if less than 5 mm. These injuries are repaired in two layers with 2-0 silk sutures in a running style. The first layer should include the full thickness of the small bowel mucosa. The second imbricating layer should include the bowel wall musculature and serosa. The orientation of the closure should be perpendicular to the long axis of the bowel lumen in order to minimize the reduction of the lumen diameter. Small bowel defects less than 5 mm should be repaired by resection and reanastomosis. Once one small bowel injury is identified, an exhaustive search for additional injuries should be undertaken. The bowel should be inspected from the terminal ileum to the ligament of Treitz to rule out additional sites of injury.

Large bowel injuries can typically be closed primarily if the defect is 1 cm or less. The orientation of the closure is less important for large bowel defects because of the inherently larger lumen and less risk of lumen stricture. The closure is accomplished in a fashion similar to that described above for the closure of a small bowel injury. Large bowel defects greater than 1 cm should be repaired with resection of the injured segment and reanastomosis. We recommend following with drain placement and genitourinary or gastrointestinal repair. Unless otherwise indicated, the drain is typically left in place until the patient is discharged. Repair failures can occasionally be identified by examining drain contents prior to the onset of clinical symptoms and early intervention can improve patient outcomes.

 PITFALLS

- Other authors have made special mention that Sampson artery is inconsequential in most gynecologic procedures but can result in significant bleeding if not properly secured and ligated in a peripartum hysterectomy.
- Care must be taken not to disrupt the venous sinuses that are present laterally in the uterine vesicular pillars as these veins are usually very congested, and given their close proximity to the ureters, bleeding from them can be difficult to safely control.

🛡 SAFEGUARDS

- In an ideal situation, the surgeon's hand is then placed around the lower uterine segment and the distal end of the cervix is palpated, a process which marks the distal end of the bladder dissection and the limits of the cardinal ligament transection. However, the cervix in a peripartum hysterectomy is often difficult to palpate accurately, especially if it is significantly effaced with prior labor.
- All pedicles are then reexamined for hemostasis. Bleeding at the lateral margins of the vaginal cuff can be controlled with suture ligatures but caution must be taken to avoid the ureter at this location. Of note, we prefer to leave all suture ends to be marginally longer than normal. This allows for pedicle identification in cases necessitating surgical re-exploration to be a useful practice.
- The increased size of peripartum uterine and ovarian vessels and their branches as well as the significant edema present in surrounding tissue can result in slippage of the clamped vascular pedicle or shearing of clamped vessels resulting in significant hemorrhage. In an effort to decrease these risks, we have begun to utilize the use of a vessel-sealing device to secure the majority of vascular pedicles when performing a peripartum hysterectomy.
- Using the vessel-sealing device, the area of bladder containing ectopic placental tissue is excised with care taken to avoid the bladder trigone and ureteral orifices. We find that this technique dramatically reduces blood loss in cases of placenta percreta.
- The most important aspect of managing a genitourinary injury is accurately identifying the injury itself; therefore, every effort should be made to continuously evaluate the bladder and ureters during a peripartum hysterectomy to minimize the risk of injury and to maximize to chances of identifying an injury should one occur.

REFERENCES

1. Cahill A, et al. Obstetric Care Consensus No. 7: Placenta Accreta Spectrum. *Obstet Gynecol.* 2018;132(6):e259-e275. doi:10.1097/AOG.0000000000002983.
2. Fitzpatrick KE, Sellers S, Spark P, Kurinczuk JJ, Brocklehurst P, Knight M. The management and outcomes of placenta accreta, increta, and percreta in the UK: a population-based descriptive study. *Br J Obstet Gynecol.* 2014;121(1):62-70; discussion -1.
3. Abudhamad A. Morbidly adhered placenta. *Semin Perinatol.* 2013;37(5):359-364. doi:10.1053/j.semperi.2013.06.014.
4. Flood KM, Said S, Geary M, Robson M, Fitzpatrick C, Malone FD. Changing trends in peripartum hysterectomy over the last 4 decades. *Am J Obstet Gynecol.* 2009;200(6):632.e1-632.e6.
5. Glaze S, Ekwalanga P, Roberts G, Lange I, Birch C, Rosengarten A. Peripartum hysterectomy: 1999 to 2006. *Obstet Gynecol.* 2008;111(3):732-738.
6. Rossi AC, Lee RH, Chmait RH. Emergency postpartum hysterectomy for uncontrolled postpartum bleeding: a systematic review. *Obstet Gynecol.* 2010;115(3):637-644.
7. Bodelon C, Bernabe-Ortiz A, Schiff MA, Reed SD. Factors associated with peripartum hysterectomy. *Obstet Gynecol.* 2009;114(1):115-123.
8. Belfort MA, Shamshiraz AA, Fox K. Minimizing blood loss at Cesarean-hysterectomy for placenta previa percreta. *Am J Obstet Gynecol.* 2017;216(1):78 e1-e2.
9. Baskett TF. Peripartum hysterectomy. In: Arulkumaran S, Karoshi M, Keith LG, Lalonde AB, B-Lynch C, eds. *Postpartum Hemorrhage.* 2nd ed. London, UK: Sapiens Publishing; 2012.
10. Swaim LS, Dildy GAIII. Surgical management of obstetrical emergencies. In: Macones GA, Wiley B, eds. *Management of Labor & Delivery.* 2nd ed. Oxford, UK; 2016.

11. Cunningham GA, Leveno KJ, Bloom SL, et al, eds. *Williams Obstetrics*. 25th ed. New York, NY, USA: McGraw Hill; 2018.

12. Castellano T, Zerden M, Marsh L, Boggess K. Risks and benefits of salpingectomy at the time of sterilization. *Obstet Gynecol Surv*. 2017;72(11):663-668.

13. Duncan JR, Jones HL, Hoffer SO, Schenone MH, Mari G. Bilateral salpingectomy versus bilateral partial salpingectomy during Cesarean delivery. *Int J Womens Health*. 2018;10:649-653.

14. Ganer Herman H, Gluck O, Keidar R, Kerner R, Kovo M, Levran D. Ovarian reserve following Cesarean section with salpingectomy vs tubal ligation: a randomized trial. *Am J Obstet Gynecol*. 2017;217(4):472.e1-472.e6.

15. Druzijanic N, Pogorelic Z, Perko Z, Mrklic I, Tomic S. Comparison of lateral thermal damage of the human peritoneum using monopolar diathermy, harmonic scalpel and LigaSure. *Can J Surg*. 2012;55(5):317-321.

16. Gibbs S, Widelock T, Elkattah R, Depasquale S. Additional uses of a vaginal fornices delineator. *Am J Obstet Gynecol*. 2015;213(3):433.e1-433.e3.

17. Van den Akker T, Brobbel C, Dekkers OM, Bloemenkamp KW. Prevalence, indications, risk Indicators, and outcomes of emergency peripartum hysterectomy worldwide: a systematic review and meta-analysis. *Obstet Gynecol*. 2016;128(6):1281-1294.

18. Kwee A, Bots ML, Visser GH, Bruinse HW. Emergency peripartum hysterectomy: a prospective study in The Netherlands. *Eur J Obstet Gynecol Reprod Biol*. 2006;124(2):187-192.

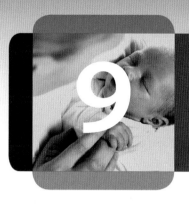

9 Urologic and Gastrointestinal Injuries

Kristy K. Ward

While urological and bowel injuries are very rare during caesarian section, a busy obstetrician will encounter a few such injuries and should be prepared. It is most important that the obstetric surgeon can quickly identify these injuries intraoperatively and call for assistance from a specialist. Intraoperative diagnosis and treatment are the key to quick patient recovery.

All obstetricians are familiar with the intimate relationship of the bladder and distal ureters to the uterus (Figure 9-1). While the pregnant uterus usually holds the bowel out of the operative field, adhesive disease can pull the bowel into the pelvis and increase the risk of injury. Fortunately, urologic and gastrointestinal injuries occur during less than 1% of cesarean deliveries.[1]

BLADDER INJURY

Bladder injury is the most common injury associated with cesarean section and is still fortunately very rare. Bladder injuries often occur at the bladder dome and are more difficult to repair if they occur at the trigone of the bladder (Figure 9-2). Incidence of bladder injury with cesarean sections is estimated to be between 0.052% and 0.8%. Repeat cesarean section is the greatest risk factor for injury. There is also increased risk of bladder injury when performing hysterotomy on a laboring uterus. Bladder injury can also occur during peritoneal entry, bladder flap creation, hysterotomy, lysis of adhesions, or during attempted hemorrhagic control.[2,3]

Assessment for Bladder Injury
- If bladder injury is suspected, the bladder must be carefully visually inspected to evaluate for any visible tears.
- If no tears are visualized, leakage should be assessed by backfilling the bladder with a colored fluid. Normal saline tinted with methylene blue can be used, but sterile baby formula is usually readily available on the OB floor and also works well.
- When performing this intraoperatively, a nurse or assistant disconnects the Foley catheter under the drape and then uses a large syringe to fill the bladder which usually requires at least 180 mL or more to see distention of the bladder. Remember to clamp the Foley tubing or the fluid will run out of the bladder.
- Leakage is confirmed when colored fluid is seen in the abdominal cavity.

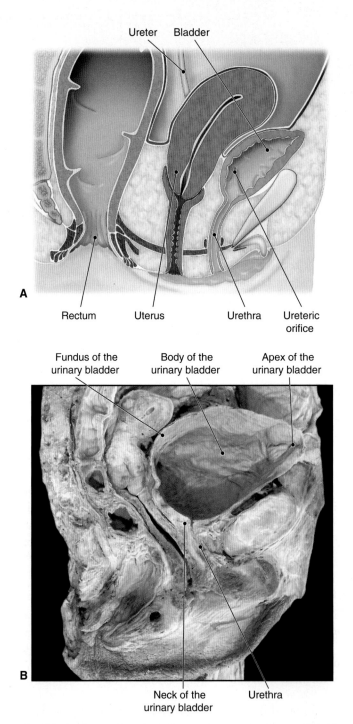

FIGURE 9-1 Female anatomy (sagittal section) showing proximity of uterus, bladder, rectum, and ureters. (Reprinted with permission from Olinger AB. *Human Gross Anatomy*. Philadelphia: Wolters Kluwer; 2016.)

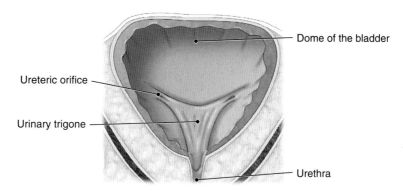

FIGURE 9-2 Parts of the urinary bladder of the female (coronal section). (Reprinted with permission from Olinger AB. *Human Gross Anatomy*. Philadelphia: Wolters Kluwer; 2016.)

Repair of Injury to the Dome of the Bladder

Injury to the dome of the bladder heals well with repair and bladder rest. The dome of the bladder can be repaired by the obstetrician with absorbable suture.

- The first layer should reapproximate the mucosa in a running fashion.
- A second imbricating layer should then be performed in the serosal layer in a running fashion.
- The bladder should be backfilled to assess leakage as described above. Any areas of leakage should be oversewn.
- The patient keeps the Foley catheter in place for 1 week, after which a voiding trial can be completed in the office.

Repair of Injury to the Trigone of the Bladder

- Injury to the trigone of the bladder requires repair by a surgeon with urologic training.
- Careful ureteral reassessment is needed before, during, and after the repair to assure patency.
- Options for ureteral evaluation include injections of intravenous endocardial mean to allow visualization of urine exhalation from the ureteral orifices or placement of ureteral stents.
- The urologist or urogynecologist may decide to place pelvic drains to evaluate for leakage. The output from the drains is tested for creatinine; if the creatinine of the fluid is greater than serum creatinine, this suggests urine is leaking into the abdomen.
- The patient retains the Foley catheter in place for 1 week.
- A voiding cystourethrogram is usually ordered prior to removing the Foley to confirm the injury has healed.

URETER INJURY

Ureteral injury should always be evaluated and repaired by a surgeon with urological training. The repair of ureteral injury is dependent on the type and location of the injury. The majority of ureteral injuries encountered during obstetric cases occur near where the uterine artery crosses the ureter. The two most common injuries result from the ureter being kinked by suture placement too close the ureter or by the ureter being

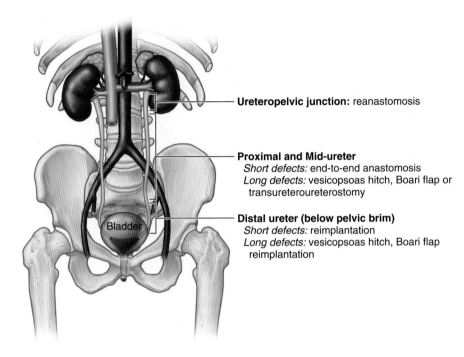

Ureteropelvic junction: reanastomosis

Proximal and Mid-ureter
Short defects: end-to-end anastomosis
Long defects: vesicopsoas hitch, Boari flap or
   transureteroureterostomy

Distal ureter (below pelvic brim)
Short defects: reimplantation
Long defects: vesicopsoas hitch, Boari flap
   reimplantation

Bladder

FIGURE 9-3 Course of the ureter and injury locations and types of repair (ureteropelvic junction, proximal and mid-ureter, distal ureter). (Reprinted with permission from Moore KL, Dalley AF, Agur AMR. *Clinically Oriented Anatomy.* 7th ed. Philadelphia: Wolters Kluwer; 2014.)

mistakenly tied in an attempt to ligate the uterine artery. The method of repair for ureteral injury depends on the level of the injury (below the pelvic brim, mid-ureter, or proximal ureter) (Figure 9-3). Repair techniques include reimplantation, end-to-end reanastomosis, and anastomosis of the injured ureter to the normal one.

Assessment for Ureteral Injury

- The obstetrician should carefully trace the ureter along its course to identify a site of injury, and cystoscopy should be performed to see if there is reflux from the ureteral orifices bilaterally.
- Intravenous dye or mannitol distension of the bladder should be used for better visualization of the ureteral efflux.
- If the bladder is filled with colored fluid prior to cystoscope insertion, irrigation should be performed.[4]
- Indigo carmine was one of the most commonly used intravenous materials to evaluate ureteral flow but is no longer manufactured. Intravenous sodium fluorescein will adequately tint the urine to allow visualization of efflux.

Procedure for Repair of Injury to Ureter

- If the suture does not involve the ureter and can be removed, the suture should be removed and cystoscopy performed to evaluate ureteral efflux.
- Note that crush-and-burn injuries of the ureter may take a few days before showing disturbances in urine flow. If there is concern, a urologic specialist should be consulted to evaluate for stent placement.

- If still no ureteral efflux, consult urology or urogynecology to attempt to insert a stent. If the stent can be passed, the urologist will advise on how long the stent should remain in place and if any other intervention is needed.
- If the stent cannot be inserted, further evaluation is needed to find and remove the cause of the blockage. In cases where this cannot be done (such as a hemostatic stitch in an unstable patient), the patient may need a temporary percutaneous nephrostomy with repair at a later date.

Procedure for Cut or Damaged Ureter

- If the ureter has been cut or damaged, it will likely require reimplantation. A defect that still allows adequate ureteral length may be able to be repaired with reimplantation ureteroneocystostomy alone (Figure 9-4).

Technique for Ureteroneocystostomy

- Open an incision into the bladder and insert the ureter (view Figure 9-4A).
- The ureter is transected and brought through a small cystotomy above the trigone (Figure 9-4B).
- The ureter is then tunneled between the serosa and muscularis and brought through another incision on the interior of the bladder (Figure 9-4C).
- The ureter is then sutured open inside the bladder, and a stent is placed to allow healing (Figure 9-4D).

Repair of Larger Ureteral Injury

If there is not enough ureteral length to allow repair without tension, a *Boari flap* and/or *psoas hitch* may be necessary. A Boari flap increases the bladder height to allow reimplantation of the ureter into the bladder. In the psoas hitch procedure, the bladder is mobilized to the ureter and sewn to the psoas tendon to allow tension free ureteral reanastomosis.

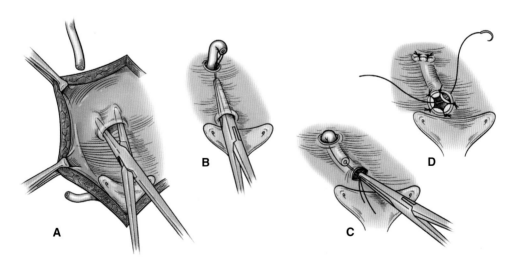

FIGURE 9-4 A-D, Ureteroneocystostomy. Injury of the ureter near the trigone may be able to be reimplanted into the bladder. A, Open an incision into the bladder and insert the ureter. B, Create a distal incision in the mucosa of the bladder and tunnel to the inserted ureter. C, Bring the ureter through the tunnel. D, Suture the ends of the ureter to the mucosa and place a stent. (Reprinted with permission from Presti JC Jr, Carroll PR. Intraoperative management of the injured ureter. In: Schrock TR, ed. *Perspectives in Colon and Rectal Surgery*. St. Louis, MO: Quality Medical Publishing; 1988. ©Thieme Medical Publishers.)

Technique for Boari Flap and Psoas Hitch

- A Boari flap involves cutting the bladder transversely across the dome and sewing it back vertically to create an extension of the top of the bladder to reach the ureter (Figure 9-5)
- A psoas hitch involves mobilizing the bladder to allow it to be repositioned and attached to the psoas, pulling it more caudally in the pelvis to reach the ureter (Figure 9-6). These two techniques of Boari flap and psoas hitch can be combined to decrease the tension on the ureter.
- A stent is placed to allow healing.[5]
- Mid-ureteral injuries can be spatulated and reapproximated performing an end-to-end ureteral reanastomosis (Figure 9-7).
- If a mid-ureteral injury cannot be reapproximated, a transureteroureterostomy can be performed whereby the proximal end of the injured ureter can be anastomosed to the ureter of the contralateral kidney (Figure 9-8).

PELVIC BRIM INJURY

Pelvic brim injuries are rare during obstetrical surgery as the usually happen when the infundibulopelvic ligament is being ligated. In the case of a pelvic brim injury, an end-to-end reanastomosis or a transureteroureterostomy is needed (Figures 9-7 and 9-8).[5]

Repair of Pelvic Brim Injury

- If the defect is small and the ends of the ureter can be brought back together without tension, both ends are spatulated and repaired with interrupted suture.
- A stent will be placed to allow healing.[5]
- If the defect is large and the ends cannot be brought back together, the proximal ureter is brought to the opposite side.
- A urethrostomy is made in the normal ureter and the injured ureter is spatulated and sewn into the urethrostomy.
- Follow-up imaging and removal of stents is dictated by the urology specialist

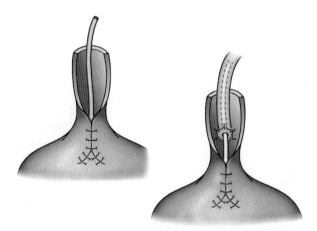

FIGURE 9-5 Boari flap. A Boari flap increases the bladder height to allow reimplantation of the ureter into the bladder. Boari flap performed using a tubularized bladder flap based on the ipsilateral superior vesical artery. (Reprinted with permission from Mulholland MW. *Greenfield's Surgery*. 6th ed. Wolters Kluwer; 2016 [Figure 26-3 View C].

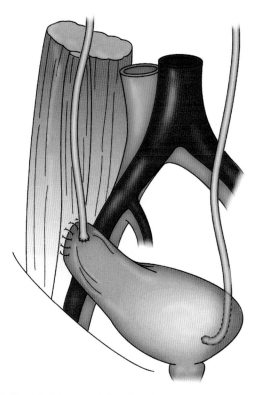

FIGURE 9-6 Psoas hitch. The bladder is mobilized to the ureter and sewn to the psoas tendon to allow tension free ureteral reanastomosis. (Reprinted with permission from Mulholland MW. *Greenfield's Surgery*. 6th ed. Wolters Kluwer; 2016 [Figure 26-3 View B].)

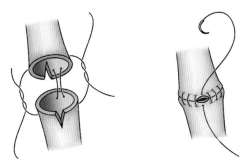

FIGURE 9-7 End-to-end ureteral reanastomosis (ureteroureterostomy) Mid-ureteral injuries can be spatulated and reapproximated. (Reprinted with permission from Mulholland MW. *Greenfield's Surgery*. 6th ed. Wolters Kluwer; 2016 [Figure 26-3 View A].)

BOWEL INJURY

Repair of bowel injuries depends on the privileges and comfort level of the surgeon. If the obstetrician is not credentialed or does not feel comfortable to undertake bowel repairs, a surgical specialist such as gynecologic oncology, general surgery, colorectal surgery, or urogynecology should be called in. Bowel injuries can be scored by the American Association for the Surgery of Trauma injury score (Table 9-1).[6]

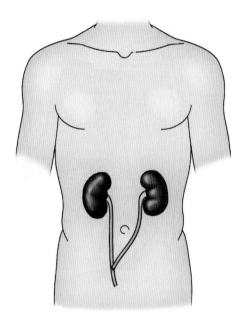

FIGURE 9-8 Transureteroureterostomy. If a mid-ureteral injury cannot be reapproximated, the proximal end of the injured ureter can be anastomosed to the ureter of the contralateral kidney. (Reprinted with permission from Mulholland MW. *Greenfield's Surgery*. 6th ed. Wolters Kluwer; 2016 [Figure 26-3 View D].)

TABLE 9-1 Small Bowel Injury Scale

Grade[a]		Description	AIS-90
I	Hematoma Laceration	Contusion or hematoma without devascularization Partial thickness, no perforation	2 2
II	Laceration	Laceration <50% of circumference	3
III	Laceration	Laceration >50% of circumference without transection	3
IV	Laceration	Transection of small bowel	4
V	Laceration Vascular	Transection of small bowel with segmental tissue loss Devascularized segment	4 4

[a]Advance one grade for multiple injuries up to grade III.

Repair of Serosal Bowel Injury

- Partial-thickness lacerations or contusions are considered a Grade 1 injury and can be easily reinforced.[6]
- Serosal injuries of the small or large bowel can be repaired with interrupted suture of 2-0 or 3-0 silk.
- Large bowel can be repaired parallel or perpendicular to the direction of the bowel whereas small bowel must be repaired perpendicular to the direction of the bowel to avoid narrowing the lumen.
- If the small bowel serosal tear is very large and cannot be repaired in a perpendicular fashion, resection and reanastomosis may be needed.[7,8]

Repair of Full-Thickness Bowel injury

Full-thickness injuries of the bowel are considered Grade 2 if less than 50% of the circumference and Grade 3 if greater than 50%. A full transection is a Grade 4 injury.[6] Grade 2 and Grade 3 injuries of the large bowel can likely be primarily repaired.

- Small bowel injuries can be repaired in one or two layers. The mucosa should be reapproximated with a 2-0 or 3-0 absorbable suture, and the serosa should be reapproximated with interrupted suture of 2-0 or 3-0 silk (Figure 9-9).
- Small bowel must be repaired perpendicular to the direction of the bowel to avoid narrowing the lumen.
- If the small bowel injury is large and cannot be repaired in a perpendicular fashion, resection and reanastomosis may be needed.[7,8]
- Large bowel can be repaired parallel or perpendicular to the direction of the bowel (Figure 9-10).

Resection and Reanastomosis of the Small Bowel (Side-to-side, Functional End-to-end)

Due to the narrow lumen of the small bowel, end-to-end anastomoses should not be performed to avoid stricture.

- To begin, a small hole should be made between the mesentery and the bowel both proximal and distal to the injured area.
- A GIA stapler is introduced in each of these holes, and the small bowel is stapled and cut (Figure 9-11)
- The injured section of bowel is removed from the mesentery with a ligation device or with suture ligation.
- The two sections of bowel are placed parallel to each other and a clamp such as an Allis is placed on the corner on the antimesenteric side of the staple line.
- The corner is removed and an arm of the GIA stapler is introduced into each lumen (view Figure 9-11A).
- The stapler is aligned so it will fire along the antimesenteric side of the small bowel (view Figure 9-11B).
- The open edge of the bowel is then closed with a TA stapler or in 2 layers with absorbable and nonabsorbable suture (view Figure 9-11C).
- If stapling devices are not available, this can be performed by hand sewing the anastomosis

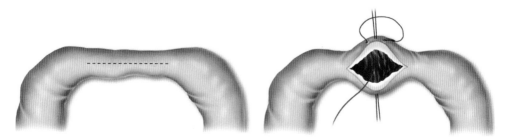

FIGURE 9-9 Small bowel serosal injury. The serosa should be reapproximated perpendicular to the bowel. (Reprinted with permission from Wexner SD, Fleshman JW. *Colon and Rectal Surgery: Abdominal Operations.* 2nd ed. Philadelphia: Wolters Kluwer; 2019.)

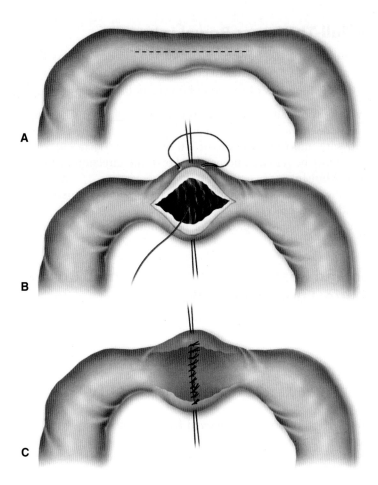

FIGURE 9-10 Small bowel full-thickness injury. The mucosa and serosa should be reapproximated in one single or two separate layers perpendicular to the bowel. (Reprinted with permission from Wexner SD, Fleshman JW. *Colon and Rectal Surgery: Abdominal Operations*. 2nd ed. Philadelphia: Wolters Kluwer; 2019.)

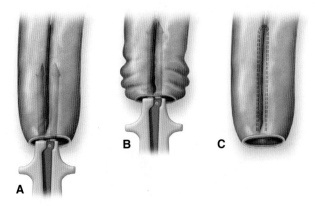

FIGURE 9-11 Side-to-side functional end-to-end anastomosis. Introduce the stapler along the antimesenteric border and fire the stapler. The sides of the small bowel are stapled together and a new lumen created allowing contents to flow in the natural direction. (Reprinted with permission from Wexner SD, Fleshman JW. *Colon and Rectal Surgery: Abdominal Operations*. 2nd ed. Philadelphia: Wolters Kluwer; 2019.)

Resection and Reanastomosis of the Large Bowel

The lumen and structure of the large bowel allows for end-to-end anastomosis without great concern for stricture, which is fortunate as the short length of the large bowel can make reanastomosis without tension difficult. In areas such as the transverse colon, side-to-side anastomosis may be able to be performed if necessary.

End-to-end Anastomosis (Figure 9-12)

- A small hole should be made between the mesentery and the bowel both proximal and distal to the injured area.
- A GIA stapler is introduced in each of these holes, and the small bowel is stapled and cut.
- The injured section of bowel is removed from the mesentery with a ligation device or with suture ligation.
- A purse string suture of prolene or nylon is placed around the proximal end with a purse string device or hand sewn.
- The suture line is cut and the anvil of the end-to-end anastomosis stapler is placed in the lumen and the purse string is tied. If the distal rectosigmoid is being repaired, the stapler side is inserted through the rectum. If the section of bowel does not allow rectal insertion, an incision is made in the bowel distal to the staple line to allow insertion of the device.
- The spike is advanced through the bowel wall as close to the staple line as possible. The anvil is attached and the device closed and fired.

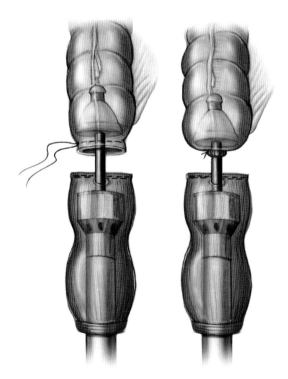

FIGURE 9-12 End-to-end anastomosis. (Reprinted with permission from Corman M, Nicholls RJ, Fazio VW, Bergamaschi R. *Corman's Colon and Rectal Surgery*. 6th ed. Wolters Kluwer Health and Pharma; 2012 [Figure 19–002].)

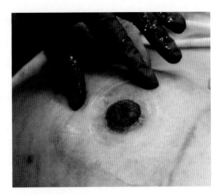

FIGURE 9-13 Colostomy stoma. Colostomy allows for diversion of the stool to outside the body. (Reprinted with permission from Lippincott Nursing Procedures, ©Wolters Kluwer Health and Pharma, 2015.)

- The device is opened to inspect the tissue removed. Two complete "donuts" should be seen. If there is a defect in the "donuts," this suggests that the staple line may not completely reapproximate the bowel.
- The staple line should be carefully inspected and any areas of concern reinforced.[8]

Colostomy or Ileostomy

The need for colostomy or ileostomy due to an injury during cesarean section is exceedingly rare. Colostomy is performed if a tension-free anastomosis cannot be performed. If the anastomosis can be completed but there is tension, a diverting colostomy can be performed to allow the anastomosis to heal. If the anastomosis cannot be performed, an end colostomy may be performed, usually with the plan to reverse the ostomy after adequate healing from the primary surgery. Ileostomies are most often performed in the case of severe small bowel obstruction where the flow must be diverted due to inability to relieve the obstruction. The portion of colon that is everted outside the body is referred to as the stoma (Figure 9-13), and this is where the ostomy bag is fitted.

Colostomies were once routinely performed if colon injury occurred on nonprepped bowel. With the advancement in antibiotic coverage, this is no longer necessary.

UNRECOGNIZED INJURIES AND POSTOPERATIVE MANAGEMENT

While most bowel and urologic injuries can be managed fairly easily intraoperatively with relatively quick patient recovery, injuries that go unrecognized intraoperatively can potentially cause severe illness in the postoperative patient.

- **Postoperative symptoms that indicate bowel or urologic injury** can include fever, abnormal laboratory results including elevated white blood cell count and creatinine, pain greater than expected, abdominal bloating, blood in the urine, or leakage from the surgical incision.
- If any of these symptoms occur, imaging such as CT scan should be performed to look for intra-abdominal collections or obvious sites of bowel or urologic extravasation.
- Fluid collections can be drained to evaluate for bowel contents or tested for creatinine to evaluate for urine (fluid creatinine > serum creatinine).

- Any concern for postoperative injury should prompt a consult with urologic or surgery specialist.
- There should be a low threshold to start broad-spectrum antibiotics as these women can quickly become septic.

 PITFALLS

- The majority of ureteral injuries encountered during obstetric cases occur near where the uterine artery crosses the ureter. The two most common ureteral injuries result from the ureter being kinked by suture placement too close the ureter or by the ureter being mistakenly tied in an attempt to ligate the uterine artery.
- Note that crush-and-burn injuries of the ureter may take a few days before showing disturbances in urine flow. If there is concern, a urologic specialist should be consulted to evaluate for stent placement.

SAFEGUARDS

- Indigo carmine was one of the most commonly used intravenous materials to evaluate ureteral flow but is no longer manufactured. Intravenous sodium fluorescein will adequately tint the urine to allow visualization of efflux.
- Colostomies were once routinely performed if colon injury occurred on nonprepped bowel. With the advancement in antibiotic coverage, this is no longer necessary.

REFERENCES

1. Hammad IA, Chauhan SP, Magann EF, Abuhamad AZ. Peripartum complications with cesarean delivery: a review of Maternal-Fetal Medicine Units Network publications. *J Matern Fetal Neonatal Med.* 2014;27(5):463.
2. Alexander JM, Leveno KJ, Rouse DJ, et al. Comparison of maternal and infant outcomes from primary cesarean delivery during the second compared with first stage of labor. National Institute of Child Health and Human Development (NICHD) Maternal-Fetal Medicine Units Network (MFMU). *Obstet Gynecol.* 2007;109(4):917.
3. Phipps MG, Watabe B, Clemons JL, Weitzen S, Myers DL. Risk factors for bladder injury during cesarean delivery. *Obstet Gynecol.* 2005;105(1):156.
4. Grimes CL, Patankar S, Ryntz T, et al. Evaluating ureteral patency in the post-indigo carmine era: a randomized controlled trial. *Am J Obstet Gynecol.* 2017;217(5):601.e1.
5. Santucci RA, Doumanian LR. Section IX. Upper urinary tract obstruction and trauma. Chapter 42: Upper urinary tract trauma. In: Wein AJ, Kavoussi NAC, Partin AW, Peters CA, eds. *Campbell-Walsh Urology.* Vol 2. 10th ed. Philadelphia: Elsevier; 2007:1169.
6. Moore EE, Cogbill TH, Malangoni MA, et al. Organ injury scaling, II: pancreas, duodenum, small bowel, colon, and rectum. *J Trauma* 1990;30:1427. doi:10.1097/00005373-199011000-00035.
7. Baggish MS, Karram MM. *Chapter 95. Small bowel repair/resection.* In: *Atlas of Pelvic Anatomy and Gynecologic Surgery.* 4th ed. Philadelphia: Elsevier; 2016:1109-1112.
8. Baggish MS, Karram MM. *Chapter 99. Colon repair/colostomy creation.* In: *Atlas of Pelvic Anatomy and Gynecologic Surgery.* 4th ed. Philadelphia: Elsevier; 2016:1123-1126.

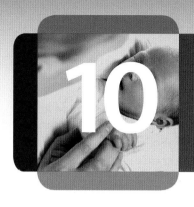

10 Postoperative Management of the Difficult Cesarean Delivery

S. Kyle Gonzales, Shae Connor, Tripp Nelson,
C. David Adair

INTRODUCTION AND HISTORICAL PERSPECTIVE

Obstetrical procedures involve the spectrum of the female genitourinary tract. This chapter focuses upon complications during and following cesarean delivery and/or cesarean hysterectomy; the underlying principles will serve the accoucheur well in the provision of complicated care to the parturient patient. Obstetric and gynecology providers participate in 3 of the top 10 surgical procedures, which include cesarean section, circumcision, and hysterectomy.[1]

Cesarean section was generally conducted in cases of maternal death in early Roman and Christian times in an effort to bring forth the unborn child and was largely, up until the early 20th century, considered a matter of last resort. Beginning with the implementation of ether as an anesthetic by Dr. Morton and antiseptic prevention by Dr. Lister, development of surgical techniques was largely advanced in the second half of the 19th century and cesarean section became a consideration. One of the first series describing cesarean delivery in France reported a 100% maternal mortality due to either hemorrhage or infection.[2] Since then, suture techniques and materials, blood transfusions, and the discovery of penicillin followed by other antibiotic developments led to a *safe* cesarean option. Today cesarean section is one of the most frequently conducted operations in the United States with almost 1.3 million procedures performed annually. Given the frequency of cesarean section and the other procedures, obstetricians who find themselves routinely conducting this surgery technique need care protocols for the expected complications that often accompany the procedure.

ENHANCED RECOVERY AFTER SURGERY GUIDELINES AND PRINCIPLES

Obstetric surgery has slowly made progress in improving postsurgical outcomes. Enhanced Recovery After Surgery (ERAS) guidelines for perioperative care have been published in colorectal, urologic, oncology, and gynecology.[1-4] Advancements in non-obstetric surgery have shown how the use of improved surgical technique can aid in reducing postoperative complications, hospital stay, recovery time, and overall health-care costs.[5,6] By using ERAS guidelines, obstetric surgery outcomes should be capable of mirroring the improvement seen in nonobstetrical outcomes. Postoperative care after a difficult cesarean section requires specific attention to detail. We discuss ERAS guidelines and address specific issues related to obstetric surgery.

POSTOPERATIVE FLUID MANAGEMENT

Generally, balanced crystalloids are preferred to 0.9% normal saline.[7] Fluids should be maintained and dosed for proper renal function. Oliguria may necessitate a fluid bolus, although gentle hydration may be required (i.e., pulmonary edema). Hypotensive patients should be managed in the proper unit, often in a critical care unit. In addition, vasopressor therapy may be indicated.

Delayed oral intake has long been a mainstay in postoperative surgical management. However, this practice has been challenged in several well-designed studies. Early oral feeds, identified as initiation of oral intake of fluid or solids within 24 hours, significantly decrease the time for bowel function to return after cesarean section without compromising gastrointestinal complications.[7,8] Studies have shown that early feeds increase nausea rates but decrease vomiting, abdominal distention, and the need for nasogastric tube use.[7] Chewing gum has also been suggested as a noninvasive measure to decrease the rate of postoperative ileus as well as return of bowel function.[7] A Cochrane review showed a reduction in the rate of ileus as well as quicker return of bowel function with limited risks or side effects, although the authors acknowledge the level of evidence is very low to low.[9] Early oral intake reduces the amount of time IV fluids are indicated. We recommend terminating IV fluids within 24 hours after surgery.

ANALGESIA

Multimodal anesthesia has been suggested to not only minimize the use of opioids but to also speed the recovery process.[10] Addressed below are several options of anesthesia that exist to meet these goals. Following a difficult cesarean delivery, the optimal approach is to combine one or more of the options.[11] Poor pain control is associated with increased postoperative complications, patient dissatisfaction, and development of chronic pain.[7]

Planned operative cases allow for the use of intrathecal agents, such as morphine sulfate. Neuroaxial opioids are more effective than systemic opioids for pain control. One benefit in a spinal injection is the quick removal of the catheter with lesser incidence of technique-related complications than epidural anesthesia.[11] Combined spinal epidural may be used for cases which are expected to be prolonged beyond routine limits. This may allow for continued anesthetic control after the operation depending on the length or severity of the case. Potential systemic side effects of neuroaxial anesthesia include hypotension, systemic toxicity, pruritis, nausea and vomiting, and respiratory depression.

General anesthesia is often required and/or desired in planned cases requiring hysterectomy, such as a known placenta accreta. Postoperative opioids should be dosed for appropriate pain control without causing respiratory depression. Opioids have long been a mainstay in postoperative pain control. This may include IV patient-controlled analgesia, periodic IV control, or oral narcotics. Patient-controlled analgesia is associated with greater patient satisfaction but included higher opioid consumption and increased complications.[12] Once able to tolerate oral analgesics, intravenous patient-controlled analgesia should be stopped and pain control transitioned to oral agents.

Oral Analgesics

Most oral analgesics are safe for women who choose to breastfeed. Acetaminophen and NSAIDs (ibuprofen and diclofenac) are considered safe for most women. The use of NSAIDs in newborns with a ductal-dependent lesion (e.g., hypoplastic left heart) should be avoided.[13] Given the concern for opioid dependence as well as passage in breast milk, we prefer to use other oral analgesics as first-line options, with oral opioids as second-line options. Due to concern for opioid passage into breast milk, we recommend providers avoid the use of codeine, hydrocodone, tramadol, and meperidine in breastfeeding women. The American Academy of Pediatrics prefers the use of morphine, hydromorphone, or butorphanol.[13]

The use of NSAIDs has been shown to decrease overall opioid use and subsequently decrease opioid-related side effects.[14] Given their benefit, NSAIDs should be considered as first-line pain control over opioids. Traditionally, it has been recommended that NSAIDs be avoided in the hypertensive postpartum patient.[15] Newer data have suggested NSAID usage may be safe for this subset of women.[16,17] The addition of IV acetaminophen with NSAIDs has been shown to improve patient satisfaction.[7]

Transversus Abdominis Plane Blocks

Transversus abdominis plane (TAP) blocks require a large volume of local anesthetic injected between muscle layers, often under ultrasound guidance. The use of TAP blocks in nonobstetric and gynecologic surgery is mounting which appears to reduce overall opioid usage. These may be considered for large surgeries or in patients where some of the above modalities are contraindicated. Multimodal pain management that decreases opioid consumption and resultant opioid-induced side effects, limited perioperative fluid administration, epidural analgesia, and transverse abdominis plane (TAP) block have all been proven to decrease rates of ileus.[18-21]

VENOUS THROMBOEMBOLISM PREVENTION

Thromboembolic events are uncommon in pregnancy but remain significantly elevated above the general population risk. An operative delivery increases the risk of a venous thromboembolism (VTE) two- to threefold above a vaginal delivery and is increased for emergent cesarean deliveries.[22,23] All women undergoing a cesarean section should have placement of pneumatic compression devices prior to incision, and we recommend continuation in the immediate postpartum period with continuation until fully ambulatory. The addition of graduated compression stockings has been shown to reduce the rate of VTE when combined with other methods.[24] Individuals with additional risk factors, such as morbid obesity, prolonged immobility, or prolonged surgery, may require anticoagulants such as low-molecular-weight heparin in combination with pneumatic compression devices.[25] When indicated, we recommend low-molecular-weight heparin 40 mg subcutaneous daily, or weight based (1 mg/kg daily) for women with a BMI >35 kg/m^2.

MOBILIZATION

Early mobilization is widely recommended among ERAS bundles across surgical specialties.[1-3,26] Benefits potentially include reduced time to return of bowel function, decreased use of opioids, and reduced risk of thromboembolism. No well-designed study has statistically proven these benefits. In the setting of a difficult cesarean section, pain and postoperative healing may inhibit mobilization for some time, but any form of mobilization, such as moving to a chair, may be beneficial. Foley catheters, IV poles, and poor pain control have been cited as barriers to mobilization, and by following an ERAS protocol, early mobilization may be more feasible.[7] We encourage mobilization within 24 hours after surgery.

FOLEY CATHETER AND DRAINS

Removal of a Foley catheter as soon as possible is recommended in the postoperative period. However, after a difficult operation, the Foley allows for proper fluid balance and maintenance. This should be removed as early as possible after a complicated delivery. Time to ambulation after cesarean decreases when the catheter is removed early.[27] Prolonged placement may be required after bladder injuries. Prophylactic antibiotics are not indicated in either of these settings, and if infection is suspected, removal or replacement is recommended. Catheter-associated infection (CAUTI) is associated with prolonged hospital stay and increased morbidity and mortality.[28]

Routine placement of drains is not indicated.[29,30] Historically, intraperitoneal drains have been placed for monitoring of bleeding or urinary leaks. As noted in gynecologic oncology literature, while drain placement has been shown to diagnose anastomotic leaks sooner, drain placement did not improve outcomes, and the lack of drainage output did not rule out an anastomotic leak.[29] If drains are indicated, then we recommend removal as early as clinically indicated.

GLUCOSE CONTROL

Perioperative hyperglycemia impairs wound healing, increases morbidity and mortality, increases hospital stay, and increases postoperative infection.[31] Physiologic response to surgery involves activation of the hypothalamic-pituitary-adrena (HPA) axis, increasing cortisol, leading to peripheral insulin resistance.[32] Therefore, when hyperglycemia is expected, we recommend routine glucose monitoring with goal values <160 to 180 mg/dL. Values may be treated with intermittent insulin injection or an insulin drip. In a randomized study in a nonobstetric setting comparing sliding scale regular insulin versus basal-bolus insulin regimen, the basal-bolus regimen showed lower mean glucose levels and significantly lower composite outcome (wound infection, pneumonia, bacteremia, respiratory failure, and acute renal failure).[33] When individuals are planned to continue basal-bolus regimens in the prolonged setting, we recommend initiating this dosing as soon as tolerated. Iatrogenic hypoglycemia is a known risk of tight control and frequent glucose monitoring is paramount.

SPECIFIC POSTOPERATIVE COMPLICATIONS

Anesthesia-Related Complications

In the United States, anesthesia complications account for approximately 2% to 3% of maternal deaths. Aspiration of gastric contents is one of the most common causes of death from general anesthesia.[34] Injury from aspiration can occur either by obstruction of the airway or chemical insult to the bronchial epithelium. Pulmonary edema, hypoxia, and rarely cardiovascular collapse and death can occur.[35] Animal studies suggest that the mechanism of death in aspiration is the release of proinflammatory cytokines, especially tumor necrosis factor (TNF)-alpha and interleukin (IL)-8.[36] The risk of aspiration is greatest during induction with endotracheal intubation and with extubation at emergence, but it can happen at any point in the postoperative period. The incidence of aspiration is three to four times higher in emergent anesthesia situations compared to elective surgeries, and the risk is particularly increased in pregnant women due to decreased lower esophageal sphincter tone.[37] Although most experts recommend rapid sequence intubation in all pregnant women, this technique is not supported by the available evidence.[38] Aspiration pneumonitis can have a fulminant course and result in respiratory compromise quickly. The primary treatment goal is respiratory support. Animal studies have shown therapeutic benefit from positive-pressure ventilation and intravenous high-molecular-weight colloids.[39,40]

Urinary Retention

Urinary retention is a common complication of both pelvic surgery and neuraxial anesthesia. Spinal anesthesia blocks both afferent and efferent nerve signals to the bladder, resulting in decreased sensation of fullness and impaired detrusor contractility.[41] During a difficult cesarean or hysterectomy, extensive dissection of the parametrial tissues may disrupt the pelvic splanchnic nerves that supply the bladder, usually resulting in a hypotonic bladder and urinary retention. An indwelling catheter, sometimes for a prolonged interval, is required to decompress the bladder and allow it to regain its normal tone.

Postdural Puncture Headache

Postdural puncture headache (PDPH), or spinal headache, is another common complication of obstetric anesthesia characterized by a positional headache that is worse when upright. The incidence of PDPH after spinal anesthesia is between 3% and 9%, depending on the type and size of needle used. More commonly, PDPH results from inadvertent puncture of the dura during placement of an epidural catheter.[42] An epidural needle has a larger diameter than a spinal needle, and PDPH is thought to result from decreased cerebrospinal fluid (CSF) pressure due to leakage of CSF through the hole in the dura. Although fewer than 6% of epidural placements are complicated by inadvertent dural puncture, the rate of PDPH in these instances is up to 88%.[43] Mild PDPH is usually treated with supportive therapy, including bed rest as needed, oral analgesics, and antiemetics. Aggressive oral and/or intravenous hydration is often encouraged in postpartum patients.[44] For patients with severe or debilitating symptoms that prevent them from carrying out activities of daily living, an epidural blood patch should be offered as definitive treatment. A blood patch involves injection of autologous blood through an epidural needle into the epidural space. Epidural blood patch has been shown to reduce the duration and intensity of PDPH compared with both conservative treatment and sham procedure in a recent systematic review based on the results of three randomized controlled trials.[45-48] The blood patch procedure usually provides immediate relief within seconds to minutes, with reported success rates between 65% and 98%.[46,49]

Spinal Epidural Hematoma and Central Nervous System Infection

Spinal epidural hematoma and central nervous system (CNS) infection are rare but potentially life-threatening complications of neuraxial anesthesia. Spinal epidural hematoma results from hemorrhage into the neuraxis. Although the incidence of spinal epidural hematoma appears to be significantly lower in obstetric patients than in other populations, the risk is increased in the setting of coagulopathy or anticoagulation therapy.[50] Hematoma is less likely with a spinal needle than with an indwelling epidural catheter.[51] The concealed nature of the bleeding necessitates a high index of suspicion in patients with progressive motor and sensory blockade and/or bladder and bowel dysfunction. CNS infection is also exceedingly rare but must be considered in patients with fever, back pain, and neurologic deficits. Epidural abscess is more likely to occur with placement of epidural catheters, whereas meningitis is more common after dural puncture. The incidence of postdural puncture meningitis after spinal anesthesia ranges from 0.2 to 1.3 per 10,000 procedures.[52] Epidural abscess following placement of epidural catheters is more common, with incidence ranging from 0.5% to 3%.[53-55] Diagnosis is confirmed with lumbar puncture or magnetic resonance imaging (MRI).

Postoperative Fever

Fever in the first few days after major surgery is common. Most early postoperative fevers are the result of inflammatory cytokine release due to the stress of surgery and will resolve spontaneously. A broad differential diagnosis should be considered, however, because fever can be a manifestation of serious complications. As with any surgical procedure, common causes of fever following obstetric surgery include surgical site infections, urinary tract infections, nosocomial pneumonia, and VTE. Surgical complications include bowel and urinary tract injuries, which are generally present early in the postoperative course with persistent fever and other signs of systemic inflammatory response.

Breast Engorgement, Infective Mastitis, Abscess

Additional etiologies that are unique to the postpartum period should also be considered. Breast engorgement may occasionally cause low-grade puerperal fever. Manual expression, pumping, and breastfeeding will relieve blocked ducts. Mastitis is characterized by a painful, erythematous, swollen breast and is estimated to occur in 2% to 10% of lactating women.[56] *Staphylococcus aureus* is the most common causative organism of infective mastitis, and empiric antibiotic therapy should include an agent with activity against *S. aureus*.[57] If untreated, mastitis can progress to breast abscess.

A tender, fluctuant breast mass with overlying cellulitis is suggestive of abscess. Ultrasound imaging can differentiate abscess from mastitis and facilitate ultrasound-guided drainage.[58]

Endomyometritis

Although the incidence has decreased with widespread use of prophylactic antibiotics, postcesarean endomyometritis remains the most common complication of cesarean delivery.[59] Prior to the modern era of prophylactic antibiotics, primary cesarean section was associated with a 30% to 40% rate of endometritis.[59] For women who receive standard antibiotic prophylaxis, the rate of endometritis is 11% for cesareans performed after the onset of labor and 1.7% for scheduled cesareans without labor.[60] Other risk factors for postpartum endometritis include bacterial vaginosis, chorioamnionitis, prolonged labor, prolonged rupture of membranes, internal fetal or uterine monitoring, meconium in the amniotic fluid, colonization with group B *Streptococcus*, manual removal of the placenta, and low socioeconomic status.[61-66] Most cases of endometritis are caused by ascending infection of the uterine cavity from cervicovaginal flora, including aerobic and anaerobic organisms.[59] Diagnosis is based on clinical findings of uterine tenderness, fever, and leukocytosis.[59] Treatment should include parental antibiotics with anaerobic activity. Although rare in the modern antibiotic era, severe complications such as pelvic abscess or necrotizing myometritis requiring hysterectomy or bacteremia and septic shock can develop. For patients who fail to respond to antibiotic therapy within 48 to 72 hours, pelvic abscess, ovarian vein thrombosis, or septic thrombophlebitis should be considered.[59] The risk of postpartum endometritis can be reduced by single-dose intravenous antibiotic prophylaxis prior to incision and vaginal preparation prior to cesarean delivery in select women. In a meta-analysis of 16 trials involving almost 5000 women, preoperative vaginal preparation with 10% povidone-iodine prior to Cesarean delivery reduced the incidence of endometritis by half in women in labor or with ruptured membranes.[67]

Septic Pelvic Thrombophletitis

It is estimated that septic pelvic thrombophlebitis (SPT) complicates 1 in 800 cesarean deliveries, a rate much greater than that of vaginal deliveries[68] (Figure 10-1). In the mid-20th century, SPT was described in a series of papers investigating women who had postpartum fever and grossly palpable intravenous thrombi and seropurulent pelvic fluid at exploratory laparotomy.[69] These early reports advocated for surgical excision or ligation of the thrombosed vessels. Now, however, SPT is largely a diagnosis of exclusion, and medical therapy is the preferred treatment. When SPT involves the ovarian vein, the presentation is usually that of an acutely ill patient with fever and abdominal pain that localizes to the affected side. Thrombosis of the gonadal veins visualized on imaging confirms the diagnosis.[70] Septic thrombophlebitis of the deep pelvic veins, however, presents much more subtly and usually cannot be detected radiographically. Often, the diagnosis is made only when a patient remains persistently febrile despite appropriate antibiotics for presumed endometritis.[71] The optimal treatment of SPT has not been well established in clinical trials due to the rarity of the diagnosis, but most experts recommend broad-spectrum parental antibiotics and systemic anticoagulation until the patient demonstrates clinical improvement and remains afebrile for

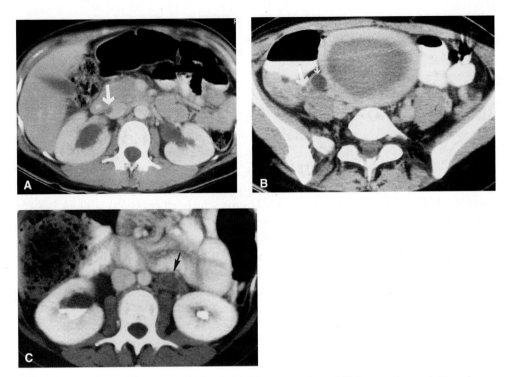

FIGURE 10-1 A-C, Ovarian vein thrombosis can be seen on these MRI images (arrows). (A and B, Reprinted with permission from Shirkhoda A. *Variants and Pitfalls in Body Imaging.* 2nd ed. Philadelphia: Wolters Kluwer; 2011. C, Reprinted with permission from Dunnick NR, Newhouse JH, Cohan RH, Maturen KE. *Genitourinary Radiology.* 6th ed. Philadelphia: Wolters Kluwer; 2018.)

48 hours.[72] Consultation with a hematologist or extended duration anticoagulation therapy may be warranted in patients with extensive thrombi or other risk factors for hypercoagulability.

Blood Transfusion Complications

The inherent risks of immunologic reaction and transmission of infectious pathogens are common to any blood product transfusion, but massive transfusion (defined as greater than 3 units of red cells in 1 hour or greater than 10 units in 24 hours) confers the risk of several unique complications.[73] Patients with obstetric hemorrhage are at increased risk for acute disseminated intravascular coagulation (DIC) due to diffuse activation and consumption of coagulation factors. Furthermore, transfusion of packed red blood cells can cause a dilutional coagulopathy due to decreased concentrations of plasma coagulation proteins and platelets.[74] Extrapolating from data in trials of severe trauma, the optimal ratio of transfused red blood cells (RBCs) to fresh frozen plasma (FFP) to platelets in patients receiving massive transfusion for obstetric hemorrhage approaches 1:1:1. Additional complications associated with massive transfusion are attributable to the large amount of citrate infused. Stored blood is anticoagulated with sodium citrate and citric acid, and accumulation of large amounts of citrate can result in metabolic alkalosis and free hypocalcemia.[75] Although the pH of stored blood is acidic, metabolism of the citrate in transfused blood generates three times the amount of bicarbonate. If the excess bicarbonate is not excreted due to renal ischemia or underlying kidney disease, metabolic alkalosis develops. Hypokalemia can then develop as potassium ions move into cells in exchange for hydrogen ions moving out of cells in response to the alkalotic extracellular fluid.[76] Conversely, hyperkalemia can result due to leakage of potassium from red blood cells that have been stored for a prolonged period of time, but this electrolyte derangement is rare without significant preexisting renal disease. Additionally, citrate binding of ionized calcium can result in a critical deficit of free calcium and lead to cardiac arrhythmias; therefore, the plasma calcium concentration must be carefully monitored following massive transfusion.[77]

Transfusion-Associated Circulatory Overload

Transfusion-associated circulatory overload (TACO) is a common transfusion reaction characterized by pulmonary edema due to hypervolemia and excess circulatory burden that presents with respiratory distress and hypoxia during or within 6 hours of a blood product transfusion. The primary risk factors for TACO are preexisting cardiac or renal dysfunction and increased volume of transfused products.[78] Although the true incidence is difficult to determine due to suspected underreporting, TACO is estimated to occur in 1% to 4% of patients receiving blood transfusions in the perioperative setting.[79] Patients who develop TACO perioperatively are more likely to require postoperative mechanical ventilation and prolonged ICU care and are at significantly increased risk of perioperative mortality compared to transfused patients who do not develop TACO.[80] As with cardiogenic pulmonary edema from other causes, treatment of TACO involves fluid mobilization with diuretics and respiratory support with supplemental oxygen or mechanical ventilation as necessary.

Transfusion-Related Acute Lung Injury

Unlike TACO, which is directly related to the volume of blood products transfused, the risk of transfusion-related acute lung injury (TRALI) is not increased with massive transfusion compared to smaller volumes of blood product replacement. Rather, TRALI is thought to be the result of extensive neutrophil activation, leading to the release of cytokines, reactive oxygen species, oxidases, and proteases that cause damage to the pulmonary microvasculature and result in inflammatory, noncardiogenic, pulmonary edema.[81] TRALI is a rare complication, occurring at a rate of approximately 1 in every 5000 transfused blood component, but it carries a significant risk of mortality.[81] In fact, TRALI is the leading cause of transfusion-related death in the United States.[82] One prospective study reported a mortality rate of 17% from TRALI.[83] In critically ill populations, the mortality rate has been reported to be as high as 47%.[84] TRALI presents as sudden-onset hypoxemic respiratory failure during or within 6 hours of a blood product transfusion. By definition, patients with TRALI will have diffuse infiltrates on chest X-ray. Although presentation may be delayed up to 6 hours, the vast majority of cases occur within minutes of initiating transfusion.[81] Compared to TACO, TRALI is more likely to be associated with fever and hypotension and less likely to respond to diuretics. If TRALI is suspected, the transfusion should be stopped immediately. Treatment is supportive and usually requires mechanical ventilation.

Respiratory Complications

Respiratory complications are common following abdominal surgery, and upper abdominal surgery carries the greatest risk. Following abdominal surgery, lung volumes are reduced in a restrictive pattern with vital capacity (VC) reduced by up to 60% and functional residual capacity (FRC) by up to 30%.[85] These changes, which are due to diaphragm dysfunction and shallow breathing, result in atelectasis and ventilation/perfusion (V/Q) mismatch. Atelectasis results in areas of the lung that are perfused, but not ventilated, leading to impaired gas exchange and hypoxemia.[86] In addition to atelectasis, cough inhibition and decreased mucociliary clearance of pulmonary secretions contribute to an increased risk of pulmonary infection and pneumonia.[87]

Acute Respiratory Distress Syndrome

Acute respiratory distress syndrome (ARDS) is an acute, diffuse, inflammatory form of pulmonary injury that presents with progressive dyspnea, increasing oxygen requirements, and alveolar infiltrate within 6 to 72 hours of an inciting event.[88] In obstetrics, the most common causes of ARDS are sepsis and profound hypotension.[35] Patients with ARDS progress through three distinct pathologic stages, an early exudative stage, a fibroproliferative stage, and finally a fibrotic stage characterized by obliteration of normal pulmonary architecture, fibrosis, and cyst formation.[89] The proportion of patients who progress to the fibrotic stage is unknown. ARDS that persists for longer than 7 days portends a poor prognosis. Reported mortality rates from ARDS vary widely and likely depend on the underlying cause.

Bowel Complications

Paralytic Ileus

Paralytic ileus is a common cause of postoperative morbidity following abdominal surgery. Although some degree of gastrointestinal (GI) dysmotility is a normal physiologic response to surgery, pathologic ileus is generally defined as obstipation and intolerance of oral intake for a prolonged period postoperatively due to nonmechanical factors that disrupt the normal propulsive force of the GI tract.[90] The pathogenesis of paralytic ileus is the result of complex interactions between inflammatory mediators and inhibitory neural transmitters. Animal studies show that the degree of intestinal manipulation at the time of surgery is directly related to both the amount of leukocyte infiltration into the intestinal muscularis and the degree of GI dysmotility; therefore, limiting manipulation of the bowels is expected to decrease the inflammatory response to surgery and prevent postoperative ileus.[91]

Incidence rates of ileus vary widely in the literature and are highly dependent on the type of surgery and the criteria used to define ileus. It is generally accepted that lower abdominal surgeries with larger incisions and greater manipulation of the bowel (e.g., colorectal and gynecologic procedures) are more likely to cause an ileus than laparoscopic surgeries with limited visceral manipulation (e.g., cholecystectomy). Other risk factors for paralytic ileus includes increased operative time, increased operative blood loss, intra-abdominal sepsis or abscess, excessive narcotic use, delayed enteral feeding, and prolonged nasogastric tube suction.[92-97] Many interventions have proven beneficial for reducing the risk of postoperative ileus. Surgical techniques that control blood loss and minimize manipulation of the bowel are also recommended.[91,92] Postoperative ileus is generally self-limited. Treatment is supportive with intravenous fluid hydration, electrolyte replacement, bowel rest, and bowel decompression as needed.

Prolonged adynamic ileus must be differentiated from obstruction. Mechanical bowel obstruction presents with the same symptoms as ileus, including abdominal distention, nausea, and vomiting. Bowel sounds may be absent or high-pitched. Therefore, presumptive ileus that does not respond to conservative management within 24 to 72 hours should prompt consideration of mechanical obstruction. The most common causes of small bowel obstruction in the postoperative setting are adhesions and hernias.[98] Imaging can differentiate ileus, which appears as diffusion intestinal distention, from obstruction, which (Figure 10-2A and B) appears as dilated proximal bowel with distal collapsed bowel and air-fluid levels.

Potential complications of small bowel obstruction include bowel ischemia, necrosis, and perforation, which can all be fatal (Figure 10-3). Early postoperative obstruction due to adhesive disease warrants an initial trial of conservation management unless there is evidence of necrosis, strangulation, or perforation. *However, failure to regain bowel function after 5 days indicates the likely need for surgical intervention. One large trial reported increased rates of mortality and prolonged hospital stays when surgical intervention was delayed longer than 5 days.*[99]

Renal Complications

Acute Kidney Injury

Acute kidney injury (AKI) in the postoperative setting usually presents with oliguria, hematuria, or an asymptomatic elevation in serum creatinine. Causes of AKI are typically classified as prerenal, intrinsic, or postrenal, depending on the portion of the renal anatomy most affected. Prerenal injury results from decreased renal perfusion seen in

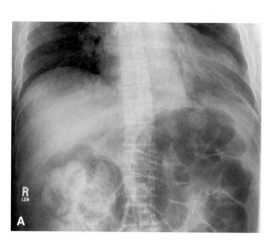
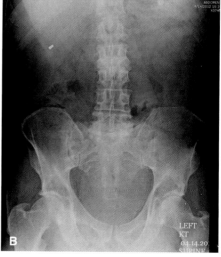

FIGURE 10-2 A and B, Radiographic demonstration of an Ileus. (A, Reprinted with permission from Jones HW, Rock JA. *Te Linde's Operative Gynecology.* 11th ed. Wolters Kluwer; 2015. B, From Cosby KS, Kendall JL. *Practical Guide to Emergency Ultra Sound.* 2nd ed. Philadelphia: Wolters Kluwer; 2014.)

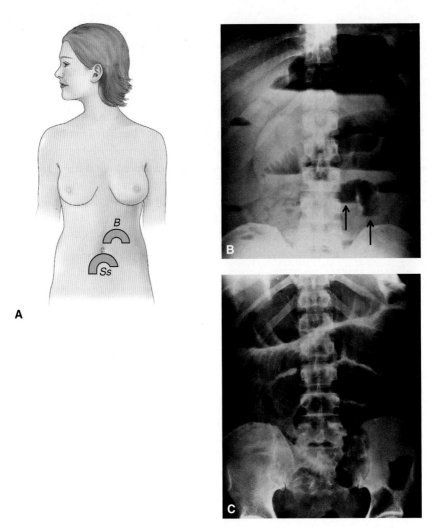

FIGURE 10-3 Bowel obstruction. A, Graphical representation of air-fluid levels, which can be a finding of bowel obstruction. B, Upright X-ray demonstrating multiple air-fluid levels related to a small bowel obstruction (arrows). C, Supine X-ray demonstrating dilated loops (arrow) of small bowel proximal to a bowel obstruction. B, balanced air-fluid levels; *Ss*, stair-step appearance air-fluid levels. (B and C, Reprinted with permission from Daffner RH, Hartman MS. *Clinical Radiology*. 4th ed. Baltimore, MD: Lippincott Williams & Wilkins; 2014.)

hypovolemic states, such as those that occur with acute hemorrhage or inadequate replacement of insensible fluid losses. Intrinsic disease can affect the renal vasculature, glomeruli, or tubulointerstitial components. Acute tubular necrosis (ATN) is the most common cause of intrinsic AKI following abdominal surgery. Postrenal disease results from obstruction anywhere in the urinary tract. Substantial decrease in glomerular filtration rate (GFR) suggests bilateral obstruction or obstruction of a single functioning kidney. The etiology of AKI can usually be established by serum and urine studies, although frequent overlap between prerenal, postrenal, and intrinsic causes exist.

Although uncommon, urinary tract injury should always be considered in the differential diagnosis of decreased urinary output and/or elevated serum creatinine in the postoperative setting, especially following a difficult cesarean or hysterectomy. The reported incidence of bladder or ureteral injury at the time of routine cesarean delivery is less than 1%, but the risk increases substantially with multiple repeat cesareans or placental abnormalities.[100] The reported incidence of urinary tract injury in cesareans complicated by morbidly adherent placenta is greater than 22%.[101,102]

Intraoperative detection of a urinary tract injury allows for immediate surgical repair and decreases postoperative morbidity; therefore, careful inspection of the urinary tract with a low threshold to perform intraoperative cystoscopy is recommended. If urinary tract injury is suspected postoperatively, expedient imaging to confirm the diagnosis should be obtained. Delayed diagnosis can lead to long-term sequelae, including fistula formation. Evaluation depends on the type of injury suspected. Renal ultrasound can diagnose hydronephrosis due to ureteral obstruction, and cystogram can detect a bladder defect. CT urography or retrograde pyelogram is usually required to localize and confirm the injury.

Wound Complications

Wound complications, including infection, seroma, hematoma, and dehiscence, are common in the obstetric population. Unscheduled cesarean deliveries confer the greatest risk of wound complication; one study reported wound complications in 28% of unscheduled cesareans.[103] Other risk factors include obesity, maternal smoking, chorioamnionitis, second-stage blood transfusion, prolonged labor or rupture of membranes, blood transfusion, anticoagulation therapy, and subcutaneous hematoma.[104,105] Multiple evidence-based interventions to decrease wound complications have been evaluated, including appropriate timing of prophylactic antibiotics, use of clippers rather than razors for hair removal, skin preparation with chlorhexidine, spontaneous removal of the placenta, closure of the subcutaneous layer if tissue depth is ≥2 cm, and subcuticular skin closure with suture rather than staples.[102,106]

Necrotizing Fasciitis

Necrotizing fasciitis is a rare but life-threatening wound complication estimated to complicate 0.18% of cesarean deliveries[107] (Figure 10-4). Early wound infections within the first 24 to 48 hours may be particularly at risk. These early infections are usually caused by group A or B beta-hemolytic streptococci and are characterized by high fever

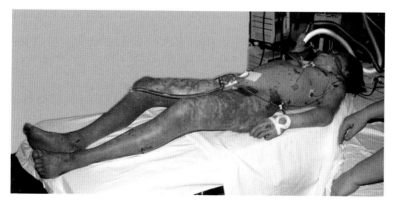

FIGURE 10-4 Necrotizing fasciitis is a rare but life-threatening wound complication estimated to complicate 0.18% of cesarean deliveries. Early wound infections within the first 24 to 48 hours may be particularly at risk. (Reprinted with permission from Staheli LT. *Fundamentals of Pediatric Orthopedics*. 5th ed. Philadelphia: Wolters Kluwer; 2016.)

and severe cellulitis.[108] Necrotizing soft-tissue infections with group A streptococci can occur at any age and in patients without other comorbidities; pregnancy and childbirth are independent risk factors.[109] A high index of suspicion must be maintained, because survival depends on prompt surgical intervention.

 PITFALL

Failure to regain bowel function after 5 days indicates the likely need for surgical intervention. One large trial reported increased rates of mortality and prolonged hospital stays when surgical intervention was delayed longer than 5 days.[99]

REFERENCES

1. Frees SK, Aning J, Black P, et al. A prospective randomized pilot study evaluating an ERAS protocol versus a standard protocol for patients treated with radical cystectomy and urinary diversion for bladder cancer. *World J Urol.* 2018;36(2):215-220.
2. Wahl TS, Goss LE, Morris MS, et al. Enhanced recovery after surgery (ERAS) eliminates racial disparities in postoperative length of stay after colorectal surgery. *Ann Surg.* 2018;268(6):1026-1035.
3. Coyle MJ, Main B, Hughes C, et al. Enhanced recovery after surgery (ERAS) for head and neck oncology patients. *Clin Otolaryngol.* 2016;41(2):118-126.
4. Nelson G, Altman AD, Nick A, et al. Guidelines for pre- and intra-operative care in gynecologic/oncology surgery: enhanced recovery after surgery (ERAS(R)) society recommendations–part I. *Gynecol Oncol.* 2016;140(2):313-322.
5. Wilmore DW, Kehlet H. Management of patients in fast track surgery. *Br Med J.* 2001;322(7284):473-476.
6. Wilson RD, Caughey AB, Wood SL, et al. Guidelines for antenatal and preoperative care in cesarean delivery: enhanced recovery after surgery society recommendations (part 1). *Am J Obstet Gynecol.* 2018;219(6):523 e521-523 e515.
7. Nelson G, Altman AD, Nick A, et al. Guidelines for postoperative care in gynecologic/oncology surgery: enhanced recovery after surgery (ERAS(R)) society recommendations–part II. *Gynecol Oncol.* 2016;140(2):323-332.
8. Hsu YY, Hung HY, Chang SC, Chang YJ. Early oral intake and gastrointestinal function after cesarean delivery: a systematic review and meta-analysis. *Obstet Gynecol.* 2013;121(6): 1327-1334.
9. Pereira Gomes Morais E, Riera R, Porfirio GJ, et al. Chewing gum for enhancing early recovery of bowel function after caesarean section. *Cochrane Database Syst Rev.* 2016;10:CD011562.
10. Kelly S, Sprague A, Fell DB, et al. Examining caesarean section rates in Canada using the Robson classification system. *J Obstet Gynaecol Can.* 2013;35(3):206-214.
11. Huang J, Cao C, Nelson G, Wilson RD. Review of enhanced recovery after surgery principles used for scheduled CD: perioperative process evaluation. *J Obstet Gynaecol Can.* 2018. doi:10.1016/j.jogc.2018.05.043.
12. Hudcova J, McNicol E, Quah C, Lau J, Carr DB. Patient controlled opioid analgesia versus conventional opioid analgesia for postoperative pain. *Cochrane Database Syst Rev.* 2006;(4):CD003348.
13. Sachs HC, Committee on Drugs. The transfer of drugs and therapeutics into human breast milk: an update on selected topics. *Pediatrics.* 2013;132(3):e796-e809.
14. McDaid C, Maund E, Rice S, Wright K, Jenkins B, Woolacott N. Paracetamol and selective and non-selective non-steroidal anti-inflammatory drugs (NSAIDs) for the reduction of morphine-related side effects after major surgery: a systematic review. *Health Technol Assess.* 2010;14(17):1-153, iii-iv.
15. American College of Obstetrician and Gynecologists, Task Force on Hypertension in Pregnancy. Hypertension in pregnancy. Report of the American College of Obstetricians and Gynecologists' task force on hypertension in pregnancy. *Obstet Gynecol.* 2013;122(5):1122-1131.

16. Viteri OA, England JA, Alrais MA, et al. Association of nonsteroidal antiinflammatory drugs and postpartum hypertension in women with preeclampsia with severe features. *Obstet Gynecol.* 2017;130(4):830-835.

17. Blue NR, Murray-Krezan C, Drake-Lavelle S, et al. Effect of ibuprofen vs acetaminophen on postpartum hypertension in preeclampsia with severe features: a double-masked, randomized controlled trial. *Am J Obstet Gynecol.* 2018;218(6):616 e611-616 e618.

18. Liu SS, Wu CL. Effect of postoperative analgesia on major postoperative complications: a systematic update of the evidence. *Anesth Analg.* 2007;104(3):689-702.

19. Torgeson M, Kileny J, Pfeifer C, Narkiewicz L, Obi S. Conventional epidural vs transversus abdominis plane block with liposomal bupivacaine: a randomized trial in colorectal surgery. *J Am Coll Surg.* 2018;227(1):78-83.

20. Helander EM, Webb MP, Bias M, Whang EE, Kaye AD, Urman RD. A comparison of multimodal analgesic approaches in institutional enhanced recovery after surgery protocols for colorectal surgery: pharmacological agents. *J Laparoendosc Adv Surg Tech.* 2017;27(9):903-908.

21. Nisanevich V, Felsenstein I, Almogy G, Weissman C, Einav S, Matot I. Effect of intraoperative fluid management on outcome after intraabdominal surgery. *Anesthesiology.* 2005;103(1):25-32.

22. Blondon M, Casini A, Hoppe KK, Boehlen F, Righini M, Smith NL. Risks of venous thromboembolism after cesarean sections: a meta-analysis. *Chest.* 2016;150(3):572-596.

23. Landon MB, Hauth JC, Leveno KJ, et al. Maternal and perinatal outcomes associated with a trial of labor after prior cesarean delivery. *N Engl J Med.* 2004;351(25):2581-2589.

24. Sachdeva A, Dalton M, Amaragiri SV, Lees T. Graduated compression stockings for prevention of deep vein thrombosis. *Cochrane Database Syst Rev.* 2014;(12):CD001484.

25. ACOG Practice Bulletin No. 196 Summary. Thromboembolism in pregnancy. *Obstet Gynecol.* 2018;132(1):243-248.

26. Nelson G, Kiyang LN, Chuck A, Thanh NX, Gramlich LM. Cost impact analysis of enhanced recovery after surgery program implementation in Alberta colon cancer patients. *Curr Oncol.* 2016;23(3):e221-e227.

27. Onile TG, Kuti O, Orji EO, Ogunniyi SO. A prospective randomized clinical trial of urethral catheter removal following elective cesarean delivery. *Int J Gynaecol Obstet.* 2008;102(3):267-270.

28. Klevens RM, Edwards JR, Richards CL Jr, et al. Estimating health care-associated infections and deaths in U.S. hospitals, 2002. *Public Health Rep.* 2007;122(2):160-166.

29. Kalogera E, Dowdy SC, Mariani A, Aletti G, Bakkum-Gamez JN, Cliby WA. Utility of closed suction pelvic drains at time of large bowel resection for ovarian cancer. *Gynecol Oncol.* 2012;126(3):391-396.

30. Karliczek A, Jesus EC, Matos D, Castro AA, Atallah AN, Wiggers T. Drainage or nondrainage in elective colorectal anastomosis: a systematic review and meta-analysis. *Colorectal Dis.* 2006;8(4):259-265.

31. Kiran RP, Turina M, Hammel J, Fazio V. The clinical significance of an elevated postoperative glucose value in nondiabetic patients after colorectal surgery: evidence for the need for tight glucose control? *Ann Surg.* 2013;258(4):599-604; discussion 604-605.

32. Desborough JP. The stress response to trauma and surgery. *Br J Anaesth.* 2000;85(1):109-117.

33. Umpierrez GE, Smiley D, Jacobs S, et al. Randomized study of basal-bolus insulin therapy in the inpatient management of patients with type 2 diabetes undergoing general surgery (RABBIT 2 surgery). *Diabetes Care.* 2011;34(2):256-261.

34. Li G, Warner M, Lang BH, Huang L, Sun LS. Epidemiology of anesthesia-related mortality in the United States, 1999-2005. *Anesthesiology.* 2009;110(4):759-765.

35. Hawkins JL, Chang J, Palmer SK, Gibbs CP, Callaghan WM. Anesthesia-related maternal mortality in the United States: 1979-2002. *Obstet Gynecol.* 2011;117(1):69-74.

36. Folkesson HG, Matthay MA, Hebert CA, Broaddus VC. Acid aspiration-induced lung injury in rabbits is mediated by interleukin-8-dependent mechanisms. *J Clin Invest.* 1995;96(1):107-116.

37. Janda M, Scheeren TW, Noldge-Schomburg GF. Management of pulmonary aspiration. *Best Pract Res Clin Anaesthesiol.* 2006;20(3):409-427.

38. Neilipovitz DT, Crosby ET. No evidence for decreased incidence of aspiration after rapid sequence induction. *Can J Anaesth.* 2007;54(9):748-764.

39. Cameron JL, Sebor J, Anderson RP, Zuidema GD. Aspiration pneumonia. Results of treatment by positive-pressure ventilation in dogs. *J Surg Res.* 1968;8(9):447-457.

40. Broe PJ, Toung TJ, Permutt S, Cameron JL. Aspiration pneumonia: treatment with pulmonary vasodilators. *Surgery.* 1983;94(1):95-99.

41. Baldini G, Bagry H, Aprikian A, Carli F. Postoperative urinary retention: anesthetic and perioperative considerations. *Anesthesiology*. 2009;110(5):1139-1157.

42. ACOG Committee Opinion No. 578: elective surgery and patient choice. *Obstet Gynecol*. 2013;122(5):1134-1138.

43. Sprigge JS, Harper SJ. Accidental dural puncture and post dural puncture headache in obstetric anaesthesia: presentation and management: a 23-year survey in a district general hospital. *Anaesthesia*. 2008;63(1):36-43.

44. Harrington BE, Schmitt AM. Meningeal (postdural) puncture headache, unintentional dural puncture, and the epidural blood patch: a national survey of United States practice. *Reg Anesth Pain Med*. 2009;34(5):430-437.

45. Boonmak P, Boonmak S. Epidural blood patching for preventing and treating post-dural puncture headache. *Cochrane Database Syst Rev*. 2010;(1):CD001791.

46. van Kooten F, Oedit R, Bakker SL, Dippel DW. Epidural blood patch in post dural puncture headache: a randomised, observer-blind, controlled clinical trial. *J Neurol Neurosurg Psychiatry*. 2008;79(5):553-558.

47. Seebacher J, Ribeiro V, LeGuillou JL, et al. Epidural blood patch in the treatment of post dural puncture headache: a double blind study. *Headache*. 1989;29(10):630-632.

48. Sandesc D, Lupei MI, Sirbu C, Plavat C, Bedreag O, Vernic C. Conventional treatment or epidural blood patch for the treatment of different etiologies of post dural puncture headache. *Acta Anaesthesiol Belg*. 2005;56(3):265-269.

49. Banks S, Paech M, Gurrin L. An audit of epidural blood patch after accidental dural puncture with a Tuohy needle in obstetric patients. *Int J Obstet Anesth*. 2001;10(3):172-176.

50. Rosero EB, Joshi GP. Nationwide incidence of serious complications of epidural analgesia in the United States. *Acta Anaesthesiol Scand*. 2016;60(6):810-820.

51. Vandermeulen EP, Van Aken H, Vermylen J. Anticoagulants and spinal-epidural anesthesia. *Anesth Analg*. 1994;79(6):1165-1177.

52. Baer ET. Post-dural puncture bacterial meningitis. *Anesthesiology*. 2006;105(2):381-393.

53. Cook TM, Counsell D, Wildsmith JA. Royal College of Anaesthetists Third National Audit P. Major complications of central neuraxial block: report on the Third National Audit Project of the Royal College of Anaesthetists. *Br J Anaesth*. 2009;102(2):179-190.

54. Sethna NF, Clendenin D, Athiraman U, Solodiuk J, Rodriguez DP, Zurakowski D. Incidence of epidural catheter-associated infections after continuous epidural analgesia in children. *Anesthesiology*. 2010;113(1):224-232.

55. Reynolds F. Neurological infections after neuraxial anesthesia. *Anesthesiol Clin*. 2008;26(1):23-52, v.

56. Committee on Health Care for Underserved Women ACoO. Gynecologists. ACOG Committee Opinion No. 361: breastfeeding: maternal and infant aspects. *Obstet Gynecol*. 2007;109(2 Pt 1):479-480.

57. Dixon JM, Khan LR. Treatment of breast infection. *Br Med J*. 2011;342:d396.

58. Dener C, Inan A. Breast abscesses in lactating women. *World J Surg*. 2003;27(2):130-133.

59. Duff P, Birsner M. Maternal and perinatal infection in pregnancy: bacterial. In: Gabbe SG, Niebyl JR, Simpson JL, et al, eds. *Obstetrics: Normal and Problem Pregnancies*. 7th ed. Philadelphia, PA: Elsevier; 2017:chap 54.

60. Smaill FM, Gyte GM. Antibiotic prophylaxis versus no prophylaxis for preventing infection after cesarean section. *Cochrane Database Syst Rev*. 2010;(1):CD007482.

61. D'Angelo LJ, Sokol RJ. Time-related peripartum determinants of postpartum morbidity. *Obstet Gynecol*. 1980;55(3):319-323.

62. Bobitt JR, Ledger WJ. Amniotic fluid analysis. Its role in maternal neonatal infection. *Obstet Gynecol*. 1978;51(1):56-62.

63. Tran SH, Caughey AB, Musci TJ. Meconium-stained amniotic fluid is associated with puerperal infections. *Am J Obstet Gynecol*. 2003;189(3):746-750.

64. Wilkinson C, Enkin MW. Manual removal of placenta at caesarean section. *Cochrane Database Syst Rev*. 2000;(2):CD000130.

65. Chaim W, Bashiri A, Bar-David J, Shoham-Vardi I, Mazor M. Prevalence and clinical significance of postpartum endometritis and wound infection. *Infect Dis Obstet Gynecol*. 2000;8(2):77-82.

66. Faro S. Postpartum endometritis. *Clin Perinatol*. 2005;32(3):803-814.

67. Caissutti C, Saccone G, Zullo F, et al. Vaginal cleansing before cesarean delivery: a systematic review and meta-analysis. *Obstet Gynecol*. 2017;130(3):527-538.

68. Dotters-Katz SK, Smid MC, Grace MR, Thompson JL, Heine RP, Manuck T. Risk factors for postpartum septic pelvic thrombophlebitis: a multicenter cohort. *Am J Perinatol.* 2017;34(11):1148-1151.

69. Collins CG, Ayers WB. Suppurative pelvic thrombophlebitis. III. Surgical technique; a study of 70 patients treated by ligation of the inferior vena cava and ovarian veins. *Surgery.* 1951;30(2):319-328.

70. Brown TK, Munsick RA. Puerperal ovarian vein thrombophlebitis: a syndrome. *Am J Obstet Gynecol.* 1971;109(2):263-273.

71. Dunn LJ, Van Voorhis LW. Enigmatic fever and pelvic thrombophlebitis. Response to anticoagulants. *N Engl J Med.* 1967;276(5):265-268.

72. Garcia J, Aboujaoude R, Apuzzio J, Alvarez JR. Septic pelvic thrombophlebitis: diagnosis and management. *Infect Dis Obstet Gynecol.* 2006;2006:15614.

73. Savage SA, Sumislawski JJ, Zarzaur BL, Dutton WP, Croce MA, Fabian TC. The new metric to define large-volume hemorrhage: results of a prospective study of the critical administration threshold. *J Trauma Acute Care Surg.* 2015;78(2):224-229; discussion 229-230.

74. Miller RD, Robbins TO, Tong MJ, Barton SL. Coagulation defects associated with massive blood transfusions. *Ann Surg.* 1971;174(5):794-801.

75. Dzik WH, Kirkley SA. Citrate toxicity during massive blood transfusion. *Transfus Med Rev.* 1988;2(2):76-94.

76. Bruining HA, Boelhouwer RU, Ong GK. Unexpected hypopotassemia after multiple blood transfusions during an operation. *Neth J Surg.* 1986;38(2):48-51.

77. Howland WS, Schweizer O, Carlon GC, Goldiner PL. The cardiovascular effects of low levels of ionized calcium during massive transfusion. *Surg Gynecol Obstet.* 1977;145(4):581-586.

78. Menis M, Anderson SA, Forshee RA, et al. Transfusion-associated circulatory overload (TACO) and potential risk factors among the inpatient US elderly as recorded in medicare administrative databases during 2011. *Vox Sang.* 2014;106(2):144-152.

79. Popovsky MA, Audet AM, Andrzejewski C Jr. Transfusion-associated circulatory overload in orthopedic surgery patients: a multi-institutional study. *Immunohematology.* 1996;12(2):87-89.

80. Clifford L, Jia Q, Subramanian A, Yadav H, Schroeder DR, Kor DJ. Risk factors and clinical outcomes associated with perioperative transfusion-associated circulatory overload. *Anesthesiology.* 2017;126(3):409-418.

81. Silliman CC, Boshkov LK, Mehdizadehkashi Z, et al. Transfusion-related acute lung injury: epidemiology and a prospective analysis of etiologic factors. *Blood.* 2003;101(2):454-462.

82. Otrock ZK, Liu C, Grossman BJ. Transfusion-related acute lung injury risk mitigation: an update. *Vox Sang.* 2017;112(8):694-703.

83. Looney MR, Roubinian N, Gajic O, et al. Prospective study on the clinical course and outcomes in transfusion-related acute lung injury*. *Crit Care Med.* 2014;42(7):1676-1687.

84. Vlaar AP, Binnekade JM, Prins D, et al. Risk factors and outcome of transfusion-related acute lung injury in the critically ill: a nested case-control study. *Crit Care Med.* 2010;38(3):771-778.

85. Ford GT, Whitelaw WA, Rosenal TW, Cruse PJ, Guenter CA. Diaphragm function after upper abdominal surgery in humans. *Am Rev Respir Dis.* 1983;127(4):431-436.

86. Marshall BE, Wyche MQ Jr. Hypoxemia during and after anesthesia. *Anesthesiology.* 1972;37(2):178-209.

87. Sugimachi K, Ueo H, Natsuda Y, Kai H, Inokuchi K, Zaitsu A. Cough dynamics in oesophageal cancer: prevention of postoperative pulmonary complications. *Br J Surg.* 1982;69(12):734-736.

88. Hudson LD, Milberg JA, Anardi D, Maunder RJ. Clinical risks for development of the acute respiratory distress syndrome. *Am J Respir Crit Care Med.* 1995;151(2 Pt 1):293-301.

89. Guerin C, Bayle F, Leray V, et al. Open lung biopsy in nonresolving ARDS frequently identifies diffuse alveolar damage regardless of the severity stage and may have implications for patient management. *Intensive Care Med.* 2015;41(2):222-230.

90. Miedema BW, Johnson JO. Methods for decreasing postoperative gut dysmotility. *Lancet Oncol.* 2003;4(6):365-372.

91. Kalff JC, Schraut WH, Simmons RL, Bauer AJ. Surgical manipulation of the gut elicits an intestinal muscularis inflammatory response resulting in postsurgical ileus. *Ann Surg.* 1998;228(5):652-663.

92. Artinyan A, Nunoo-Mensah JW, Balasubramaniam S, et al. Prolonged postoperative ileus-definition, risk factors, and predictors after surgery. *World J Surg.* 2008;32(7):1495-1500.

93. Chapuis PH, Bokey L, Keshava A, et al. Risk factors for prolonged ileus after resection of colorectal cancer: an observational study of 2400 consecutive patients. *Ann Surg.* 2013;257(5):909-915.

94. Nelson R, Edwards S, Tse B. Prophylactic nasogastric decompression after abdominal surgery. *Cochrane Database Syst Rev.* 2005;(1):CD004929.

95. Abraham NS, Young JM, Solomon MJ. Meta-analysis of short-term outcomes after laparoscopic resection for colorectal cancer. *Br J Surg.* 2004;91(9):1111-1124.

96. Schwenk W, Bohm B, Haase O, Junghans T, Muller JM. Laparoscopic versus conventional colorectal resection: a prospective randomised study of postoperative ileus and early postoperative feeding. *Langenbecks Arch Surg.* 1998;383(1):49-55.

97. Mangesi L, Hofmeyr GJ. Early compared with delayed oral fluids and food after caesarean section. *Cochrane Database Syst Rev.* 2002;(3):CD003516.

98. Miller G, Boman J, Shrier I, Gordon PH. Natural history of patients with adhesive small bowel obstruction. *Br J Surg.* 2000;87(9):1240-1247.

99. Schraufnagel D, Rajaee S, Millham FH. How many sunsets? Timing of surgery in adhesive small bowel obstruction: a study of the Nationwide Inpatient Sample. *J Trauma Acute Care Surg.* 2013;74(1):181-187; discussion 187-189.

100. Salman L, Aharony S, Shmueli A, Wiznitzer A, Chen R, Gabbay-Benziv R. Urinary bladder injury during cesarean delivery: maternal outcome from a contemporary large case series. *Eur J Obstet Gynecol Reprod Biol.* 2017;213:26-30.

101. Alanwar A, Al-Sayed HM, Ibrahim AM, et al. Urinary tract injuries during cesarean section in patients with morbid placental adherence: retrospective cohort study. *J Matern Fetal Neonatal Med.* 2019;32(9):1461-1467.

102. Lau WC, Fung HY, Rogers MS. Ten years experience of caesarean and postpartum hysterectomy in a teaching hospital in Hong Kong. *Eur J Obstet Gynecol Reprod Biol.* 1997;74(2):133-137.

103. Temming LA, Raghuraman N, Carter EB, et al. Impact of evidence-based interventions on wound complications after cesarean delivery. *Am J Obstet Gynecol.* 2017;217(4):449 e441-449 e449.

104. Olsen MA, Butler AM, Willers DM, Devkota P, Gross GA, Fraser VJ. Risk factors for surgical site infection after low transverse cesarean section. *Infect Control Hosp Epidemiol.* 2008;29(6):477-484; discussion 485-476.

105. Ketcheson F, Woolcott C, Allen V, Langley JM. Risk factors for surgical site infection following Cesarean delivery: a retrospective cohort study. *CMAJ Open.* 2017;5(3):E546-E556.

106. Carter EB, Temming LA, Fowler S, et al. Evidence-based bundles and cesarean delivery surgical site infections: a systematic review and meta-analysis. *Obstet Gynecol.* 2017;130(4):735-746.

107. Sarsam SE, Elliott JP, Lam GK. Management of wound complications from cesarean delivery. *Obstet Gynecol Surv.* 2005;60(7):462-473.

108. Martens MG, Kolrud BL, Faro S, Maccato M, Hammill H. Development of wound infection or separation after Cesarean delivery. Prospective evaluation of 2,431 cases. *J Reprod Med.* 1995;40(3):171-175.

109. Stevens DL, Bryant AE. Necrotizing soft-tissue infections. *N Engl J Med.* 2017;377(23):2253-2265.

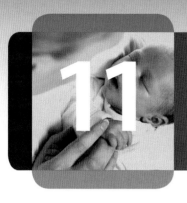

11   Anesthesia for the Difficult Cesarean Delivery

Anjum Anwar, Ted Bangert, Kristen Vanderhoef

INTRODUCTION

Providing anesthesia care for cesarean deliveries is one of the most rewarding aspects of an anesthesiologist's career. Taking part in the celebration of a new life entering the world never gets tiresome. Keeping the mother and fetus safe leading up to delivery and taking care of mom after delivery are the anesthesiologist's primary concerns. Unfortunately, the growing obesity epidemic and increased number of cesarean deliveries leading to abnormal placentation make this task increasingly difficult. This chapter will focus on these two groups but will also touch upon higher order repeat cesarean deliveries and the pertinent anesthesia concerns. The common theme of any difficult delivery is the need for individualized care involving optimal communication across disciplines.

Providing anesthesia for the difficult cesarean section (CS) patient requires preparation and a multidisciplinary team approach. Inclusion of the anesthesia team early in pregnancy, when possible, is of utmost importance. Together we can strive to provide the best care possible for our most challenging patients.

PHYSIOLOGICAL AND ANATOMICAL CHANGES IN HEALTHY PARTURIENTS

There are changes to nearly every organ system in healthy women during pregnancy. The respiratory system sees an increase in minute ventilation, alveolar ventilation, tidal volume, and respiratory rate with pregnancy (Figure 11-1). Cardiovascular changes include increases in blood volume, plasma volume, cardiac output, stroke volume, and heart rate. Plasma volume increases more than red cell volume leading to a physiologic anemia. There is a decrease in mean arterial blood pressure. For the nervous system, there is importantly a decrease in anesthetic requirements; this includes local anesthetics for standard vaginal delivery or CS as well as inhalational agents should general anesthesia be required. The gastrointestinal system has an increase in gastrointestinal reflux disease secondary to increased volume and acidity of gastric contents as well as diminished lower esophageal sphincter tone, increasing the risk of pulmonary aspiration.[1] The kidneys present with an increase in glomerular filtration rate and a subsequent decrease in creatinine. Levels of nearly all coagulation factors also increase during pregnancy, causing a hypercoagulable state.

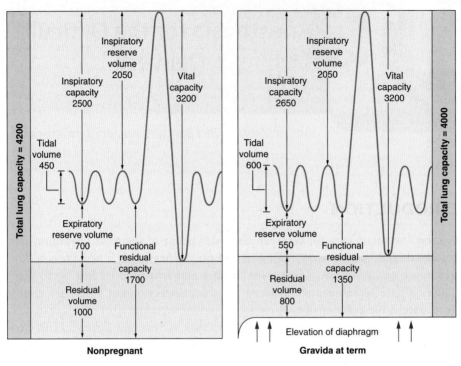

FIGURE 11-1 Normal lung volume changes in pregnancy. (From Suresh M. *Shnider and Levinson's Anesthesia for Obstetrics*. 5th ed. Philadelphia: Wolters Kluwer; 2013.)

ANESTHESIA CHALLENGES FOR THE HEALTHY PARTURIENT

There are factors complicating the anesthetic plan for any pregnant patient. First, parturients are more likely to have an airway that is more difficult for endotracheal intubation. Also, pregnant patients greater than 20 weeks estimated gestational age are considered to have a full stomach, regardless of timing of last oral intake. Details about the airway and gastrointestinal tract are discussed later in the chapter. Pregnant women are more at risk for failed intubation and aspiration due to these airway and gastrointestinal changes, and it is due to those risks that neuraxial anesthesia is almost always preferable over general anesthesia. Intraoperatively, the obstetric anesthesiologist must always be aware of, among other complications, the potential for hypotension after neuraxial anesthesia as well as intraoperative blood loss. Postoperatively, some of the more common complications requiring vigilance include pain, nausea, and hypovolemia.

MORBID OBESITY

Morbid obesity in pregnancy has deleterious effects on multiple organ systems. Morbidly obese patients present with many challenges, and these patients should have a consultation with an anesthesiologist early in their pregnancy. In the United States in 2015 to 2016, the prevalence of obesity was 39.8% affecting a total of 93.3 million adults.[2] The prevalence of obesity in pregnancy is similar; approximately, 24.8% of women delivering live-born infants in 2014 were obese before becoming pregnant.[3] In

TABLE 11-1 Physiological and Anatomical Changes in a Morbidly Obese Parturient

Factors That Complicate Cesarean Deliveries in Morbidly Obese Patients
• Difficult airway
• Obstructive sleep apnea
• Reduced functional residual capacity
• Exaggerated aortocaval compression
• Increase chance of aspiration
• Difficult placement of neuraxial anesthetic
• Difficult IV access
• Increased maternal mortality

addition to the complications mentioned below, obesity also increases the maternal risk of venous thromboembolism, preeclampsia, gestational diabetes, wound breakdown, and infection.[4] These patients generally present with other chronic non–pregnancy-related comorbidities as well, such as hypertension, hyperlipidemia, and obstructive sleep apnea (OSA) (Table 11-1). Unfortunately, these patients have a higher chance of requiring cesarean delivery, as well as higher risk of requiring emergent cesarean delivery. Several studies have shown that increasing BMI increases cesarean section rates.[4]

THE OBSTETRIC DIFFICULT AIRWAY

The pregnant airway can be precarious for a number of reasons. The physiology of pregnancy causes venous engorgement as well as upper airway edema, which makes tracheal intubation more difficult. Enlarged breasts can hinder laryngoscope placement. A combination of decreased functional residual capacity (FRC) and increased oxygen consumption results in a decreased time to oxygen desaturation with induction of anesthesia (Figure 11-2), making rapid control of the airway

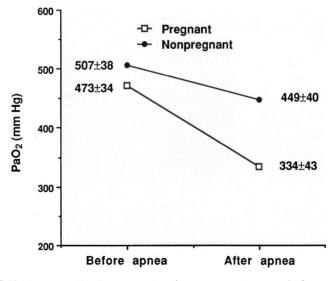

FIGURE 11-2 Patient oxygenation in pregnant and nonpregnant women before and after apnea. (From Suresh M. *Shnider and Levinson's Anesthesia for Obstetrics*. 5th ed. Philadelphia: Wolters Kluwer; 2013.)

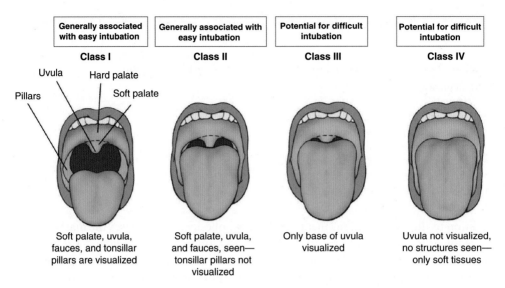

Generally associated with easy intubation	Generally associated with easy intubation	Potential for difficult intubation	Potential for difficult intubation
Class I	**Class II**	**Class III**	**Class IV**
Soft palate, uvula, fauces, and tonsillar pillars are visualized	Soft palate, uvula, and fauces, seen— tonsillar pillars not visualized	Only base of uvula visualized	Uvula not visualized, no structures seen— only soft tissues

Uvula · Hard palate · Soft palate · Pillars

FIGURE 11-3 Mallampati score is used to help predict the difficulty of intubation. A class I airway in general predicts the smallest chance of difficult intubation, and class IV airways in general give the highest likelihood of difficult intubation. (From Suresh M. *Shnider and Levinson's Anesthesia for Obstetrics.* 5th ed. Philadelphia: Wolters Kluwer; 2013.)

essential. A thorough physical examination of the airway includes Mallampati score (Figure 11-3), the patient's ability to protrude the jaw anteriorly (Figure 11-4), mouth opening, thyromental distance (Figure 11-5), neck range of motion, and the presence of loose teeth. Comorbidities such as obesity can make the airway even more challenging for intubation.

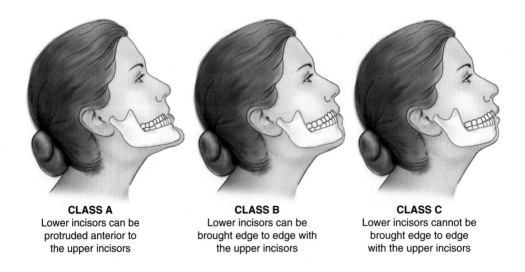

CLASS A
Lower incisors can be protruded anterior to the upper incisors

CLASS B
Lower incisors can be brought edge to edge with the upper incisors

CLASS C
Lower incisors cannot be brought edge to edge with the upper incisors

FIGURE 11-4 Airway classes defined by patient ability to protrude the jaw anteriorly. (From Suresh M. *Shnider and Levinson's Anesthesia for Obstetrics.* 5th ed. Philadelphia: Wolters Kluwer; 2013.)

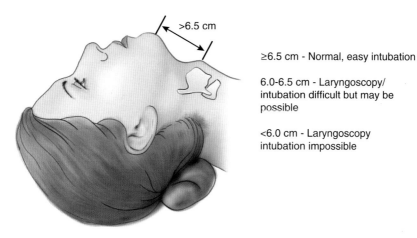

>6.5 cm

≥6.5 cm - Normal, easy intubation

6.0-6.5 cm - Laryngoscopy/
intubation difficult but may be
possible

<6.0 cm - Laryngoscopy
intubation impossible

FIGURE 11-5 Thyromental distance measurement and its implications for difficult laryngoscopy and intubation. (From Suresh M. *Shnider and Levinson's Anesthesia for Obstetrics*. 5th ed. Philadelphia: Wolters Kluwer; 2013.)

Distance Measurement and Its Implications for Difficult Laryngoscopy and Intubation

If general anesthesia is required for a cesarean delivery, adequate preoxygenation with 100% oxygen is a must. Patient positioning is also of utmost importance, with the goal of placing the patient in the "sniffing" position, see Figure 11-6. Due to the "full stomach" status of all pregnant women after 20 weeks estimated gestational age, a rapid sequence induction (RSI) is required. In this scenario, an intravenous induction agent is given immediately followed by a rapid acting paralytic without first attempting to

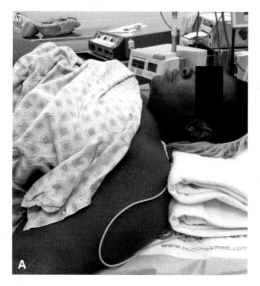
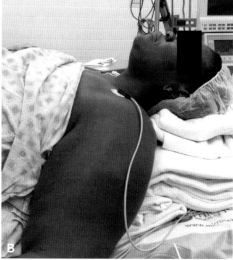

FIGURE 11-6 A "ramp" of blankets behind the shoulders and occiput of the parturient as seen before (A) and after (B) ramp placement helps place the patient in the sniffing position, which improves intubating conditions. (From Suresh M. *Shnider and Levinson's Anesthesia for Obstetrics*. 5th ed. Philadelphia: Wolters Kluwer; 2013.)

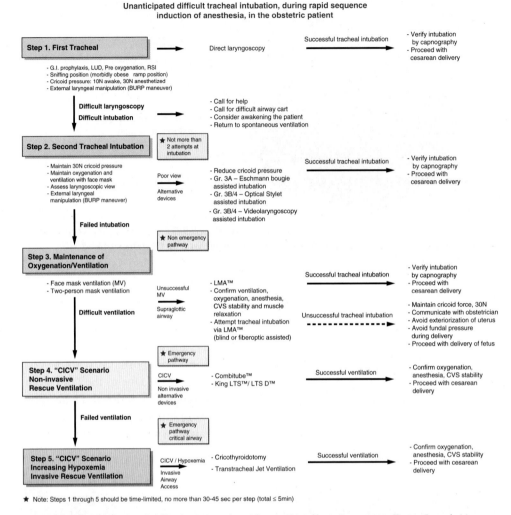

FIGURE 11-7 Unexpected difficult airway algorithm in the obstetric patient. (From Suresh M. *Shnider and Levinson's Anesthesia for Obstetrics*. 5th ed. Philadelphia: Wolters Kluwer; 2013.)

mask ventilate. If the airway is not secured quickly, PaO_2 decreases more quickly than in a nonpregnant patient (Figure 11-2) which then necessitates mask ventilation. Figure 11-7 algorithm demonstrates proper management in the difficult obstetric airway. This specific algorithm takes into account that not one, but two lives are at stake in the obstetric setting. Figure 11-8 demonstrates the importance of adhering to the difficult airway algorithm as greater than two intubation attempts can cause serious consequences. This results from tissue trauma with laryngoscope placement as well as airway edema from attempts at passing the endotracheal tube. Airway manipulation increases salivation, and bleeding may develop with airway trauma, further inhibiting the view of airway structures, making it increasingly more difficult to secure the airway.

In case of airway difficulty, it is imperative that the obstetric operating suite has emergency airway equipment readily available. This includes an assortment of endotracheal

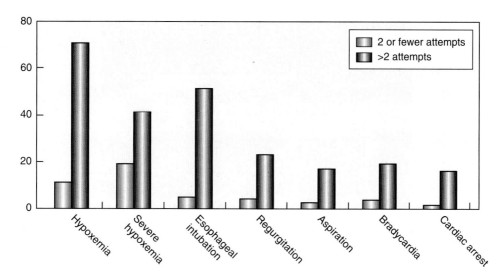

FIGURE 11-8 Visual representation demonstrating risk of increased intubation attempts. The chance of all listed potential complications increases with greater than two intubation attempts. (From Suresh M. *Shnider and Levinson's Anesthesia for Obstetrics*. 5th ed. Philadelphia: Wolters Kluwer; 2013.)

tube sizes, with focus on smaller tubes. Laryngeal mask airways (LMAs) should be available as rescue devices. A video laryngoscope is essential and frequently the intubation equipment of choice in the obstetric setting. A difficult airway cart containing a fiberoptic scope should remain on the labor and delivery floor at all times. A cricothyroidotomy kit should be placed on the difficult airway cart should a surgical airway become necessary.

Adding to the increased difficulty of any pregnant airway, obesity results in anatomical changes due to increased fat in the breasts and neck. Placing towels behind the shoulders and occiput helps align the patient into sniffing position for intubation, as seen in Figure 11-9. A short-handled laryngoscope assists in laryngoscopy when the chest and breasts are obstructing access to the airway. As stated earlier in the chapter, additional airway equipment should be available including a video-assisted laryngoscope, an LMA, a bougie, a fiberoptic bronchoscope, oral airways, and an assortment of smaller endotracheal tube sizes.

PULMONARY CHANGES

Pulmonary changes during pregnancy for the obese patient include an exaggerated decrease in FRC and increase in oxygen consumption. These changes happen in addition to the normal lung changes of pregnancy shown in Figure 11-1. Both of the two mentioned changes contribute to dramatically shortening time to oxygen desaturation in an apneic patient during intubation. Another possible consequence of changes of lung volumes is that a decrease in FRC may make the FRC smaller than closing capacity, the volume at which airways close, leading to closure of dependent airways during tidal volume respirations pictured in Figure 11-10. The airway closure then results in increased shunt (perfusion without ventilation) fraction, which then leads to hypoxemia.

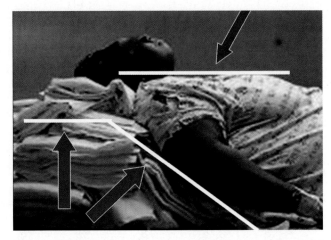

FIGURE 11-9 An obese parturient with towels placed behind her shoulders and occiput to improve laryngoscopic view. (Used with permission Robert D'Angelo, MD, Wake Forest University Baptist Medical Center, Winston-Salem, North Carolina.)

Effect of position on lung volumes

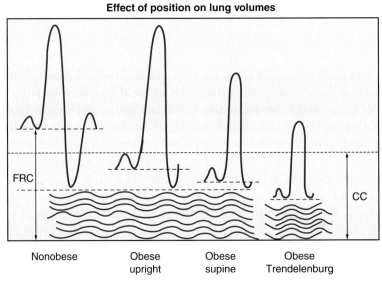

FIGURE 11-10 Lung volumes in nonobese and obese patients, further demonstrating the effects of position on lung volumes. When closing capacity (CC) is greater than functional residual capacity (FRC), alveolar closure happens during tidal volume ventilations, therefore decreasing oxygenation. This figure also demonstrates how patient positioning in the obstetric operative suite can also affect lung volumes. (From Suresh M. *Shnider and Levinson's Anesthesia for Obstetrics*. 5th ed. Philadelphia: Wolters Kluwer; 2013.)

CARDIAC CHANGES

Cardiac changes compound the difficulty of a cesarean section for an obese patient. As stated above, obese individuals are at increased risk of other medical conditions such as hypertension which can lead to cardiac changes such as left ventricular hypertrophy and impaired diastolic function. Obese young adults have a 12-fold increase in the risk of death from cardiovascular disease. This includes 25- to 34-year-olds; many parturients fall into this age group. Pregnancy further compromises cardiac status. Cardiac output may double, compared to the 35% to 45% increase for nonobese parturients.[5] In addition, aortocaval compression occurs not only from the gravid uterus but from abdominal fat as well.

GASTROINTESTINAL CHANGES

For the gastrointestinal system, the most acute concern is aspiration, for which the risk increases. A decreased lower esophageal sphincter tone and delayed gastric emptying occur for all pregnant women, and these effects are exacerbated by an increased incidence of hiatal hernias and increased intragastric pressure in obesity. An H2 antagonist, metoclopramide, and sodium citrate all decrease morbidity if aspiration occurs.

ANATOMICAL CHANGES FOR NEURAXIAL PLACEMENT

Positioning for neuraxial anesthetic placement is challenging for almost all term parturients but can be especially difficult for morbidly obese parturients at term. New positioning devices are available which can assist morbidly obese parturients with safely assuming an ideal form for placement of neuraxial anesthetics; see Figure 11-11 for an example of a neuraxial positioning device. The anatomical landmarks can be difficult to palpate, making proper positioning even more important (Figure 11-12). Ultrasound can be helpful in finding the midline and estimating the depth of the epidural space.

DIFFICULT INTRAVENOUS LINE PLACEMENT

Intravenous (IV) line placement can be very difficult in a morbidly obese parturient. Many hospitals now utilize midlines in patients with difficult peripheral access. A midline is a peripheral catheter inserted under ultrasound guidance into a larger vein than is typically utilized for IV placement. These catheters are longer than standard IV catheters, and placement into larger veins decreases the risk of phlebitis as well as infiltration.[6] If IV access proves to be difficult, an intraosseous (IO) line can be placed in an emergency.

CESAREAN SECTION ANESTHESIA FOR THE OBESE PARTURIENT

IMPORTANCE OF ANTEPARTUM CONSULTATION

Obese parturients should have a preanesthesia consultation at the start of their third trimester. This will give anesthesia providers an opportunity to obtain a detailed history and perform a physical examination as well as assess the airway. If further workup is deemed necessary, this provides plenty of time to obtain additional testing

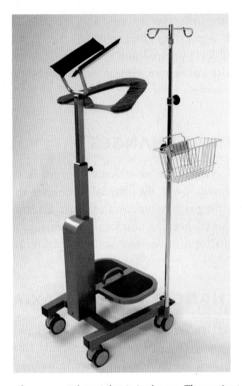

FIGURE 11-11 A positioner for neuraxial anesthesia is shown. The patient can rest her arms on the "n" shaped bottom gel pad, and she can rest her head in the top gel pads. This position helps the patient curve her back into a "C" shape, thus opening her spinal interspaces, while leaning slightly forward and maintaining her balance.

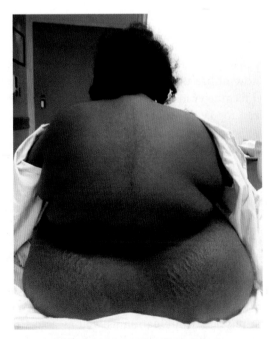

FIGURE 11-12 The back of an obese parturient. Midline and landmarks are difficult to detect. (Photo used courtesy of UF Health Jacksonville.)

and consultation with pulmonary or cardiology services. If the patient has a diagnosis of OSA, the use of continuous positive airway pressure (CPAP) should be discussed. CPAP may be required intraoperatively or postoperatively depending on severity of obstruction. Patients should be screened for OSA and sent for sleep studies, if necessary. If OSA is confirmed, CPAP should be initiated.[1] This visit also provides an opportunity for the patient to talk about her options for analgesia or anesthesia. The anesthesiologist can provide counseling on the importance of requesting an epidural early in labor to facilitate better positioning and ensure a functioning catheter as the risk of cesarean section is increased. The anesthesia options for emergency versus elective cesarean section should be discussed during this visit as well.

PREOPERATIVE PREPARATION

This is the time to prepare both the patient and operating suite for delivery. Checking the operating room table weight limit is the first step to ensure a safe delivery, followed by securing bed extensions for the operating table, if needed.

If a patient has not been seen in consult prior to surgery, the first time the anesthesia team will meet the patient would be the day of surgery. At this meeting, a history and physical examination are performed, focusing on the respiratory system, cardiac system, as well as patient airway. Discussion of anesthetic choice with the parturient preoperatively can greatly decrease anxiety pertaining to regional anesthesia. As you can see in Table 11-2 below, patient refusal is an absolute contraindication to neuraxial anesthesia; however, once risks of general anesthesia and benefits of regional anesthesia are fully explained, patients almost always agree to at least attempt regional anesthesia.

It is imperative to have adequate IV access in patients undergoing CS, necessitating the need for two well-functioning IV lines in a patient with difficult access. Prior to entering the operating room, premedication with a histamine-2 receptor antagonist and nonparticulate antacid for aspiration prophylaxis are given.

Intraoperative Neuraxial Management

Anesthesia and Medications

Surgical time is generally longer in obese patients making a combined spinal epidural (CSE) the ideal anesthetic. The patient benefits from the dense spinal block,

TABLE 11-2 Contraindications to Neuraxial Anesthesia

Absolute	Relative
Patient refusal	Mild coagulopathy
Infection at the insertion site	Severe maternal cardiac disease
Sepsis	Neurological disease
Severe coagulopathy	Severe fetal depression
Hypovolemia	

Adapted with permission from Palmer CM, D'Angelo R, et al. *Handbook of Obstetric Anesthesia*. Elsevier; 2001.

as well as an epidural catheter, which can be dosed if needed. The epidural portion of the CSE is an unproven catheter and may not function if dosing is necessary. The need to induce general anesthesia remains a possibility. Longer needle sets may be necessary to reach the subarachnoid and epidural spaces. Table 11-3 lists all the pros/cons of all choices of regional anesthesia for the obese parturient undergoing CS.[1]

The dosage for a spinal anesthetic should be injected carefully. The obstetric patient already needs lower dose of a local anesthetic due to reduced cerebrospinal fluid (CSF) volume. There should be close monitoring of hemodynamic and respiratory status after the spinal injection. Avoidance of preservative-free morphine in the spinal injection is a common practice, due to a higher risk of postoperative respiratory complications, and preservative-free morphine can increase the risk of respiratory depression in the postop period.[7] After the placement of neuraxial anesthesia and achievement of an adequate sensory deficit, the challenges continue. The patient is placed supine with a 15-degree left lateral tilt. A left lateral tilt carries greater importance in obese patients as aortocaval compression is exaggerated. Vasopressors are utilized in order to counteract the sympathectomy from spinal anesthesia. Phenylephrine is the vasopressor of choice for cesarean deliveries, due to its quick onset and titratability. Prophylactic, low-dose phenylephrine infusions (25-50 µg/min), initiated at the time of spinal injection, titrated to maternal blood pressure goals, have been shown to decrease the incidence of maternal hypotension as well as nausea/vomiting.[8]

Incision Site and Patient Positioning

Once the spinal has taken effect and final preparations are complete, the obstetric team then determines the site of incision and whether retraction of the panniculus will be necessary. If required, taping may cause additional aortocaval compression, maternal hypotension, and subsequent fetal compromise.[9] Taping the panniculus also increases diaphragmatic restriction making breathing more difficult. Placing the patient in the Trendelenburg position further compromises pulmonary function, see Figure 11-10.

TABLE 11-3 Regional Anesthesia Choices for Cesarean Delivery in the Obese Parturient

	Pros	Cons
Combined spinal epidural (CSE)	Dense subarachnoid block	Unproven epidural catheter
Epidural	Proven catheter	Less dense block
	Fewer hemodynamic changes	
Continuous spinal	Dense subarachnoid block	Theoretical risk of spinal cord penetration or spinal nerve root compression if threaded > 4 cm. Potential to be dosed as an epidural catheter causing a high spinal.
		Dural puncture could result in a post–dural puncture headache though the risk is lower in obese patients

Most term obese parturients have extreme difficulty lying flat secondary to short-ness of breath. The "ramping" discussed earlier which aids with intubation should it become necessary, also benefits patient respiration. Placing the operating table in a head up position can further assist.

Management of Other Potential Intraoperative Complications

Obese parturients are at higher risk of endometritis and wound infection; injecting prophylactic antibiotic dosing prior to skin incision is of utmost importance. The man-agement of intraoperative fluids should be monitored carefully, and euvolemia should be ensured. Obese parturients are also at higher risk for postpartum hemorrhage. Many studies have shown that blood loss during a cesarean delivery is higher in obese partu-rients.[10] Oxytocin infusion should be initiated at the time of delivery, with additional uterotonics readily available. At the conclusion of the case, safely transferring the patient from the operating table will require additional personnel. Use of an inflatable air trans-fer mattress can reduce the number of personnel needed to transfer the patient safely.

POSTOPERATIVE MANAGEMENT

The patient will spend a minimum of 2 hours in the postanesthesia care unit (PACU). One of the major problems in the postoperative period is the provision of adequate analgesia. If the CSE has been used during the surgery, use of epidural infusions for pain control is the best modality as it will reduce the need for opioids, which can cause respiratory depression, particularly in obese patients. If an epidural catheter was not placed or is not functioning, a multimodal analgesia approach would be the safest choice. This could include a combination of acetaminophen, nonsteroidal anti-inflammatory drugs (NSAIDs), and medications that target neuropathic pain, such as gabapentin. Wound infiltration with a local anesthetic at the end of surgery can also provide some relief during the immediate postoperative period.

Obese patients are at increased risk of postoperative complications. As mentioned above, these patients are at higher risk to develop postpartum hemorrhage; both the obstetricians and anesthesiologist should monitor the patient very closely. These patients can become hypoxemic in the immediate recovery period because of respira-tory depression, basal atelectasis, or even pulmonary embolism. The cardiovascular complications can include hemodynamic changes like hypertension or hypotension, myocardial infarction, and maternal death. These patients are at a higher risk to develop deep vein thrombosis (DVT) during this time. Early mobilization and DVT prophylaxis are important.

Late complications can occur in these patients including pneumonia, wound dehis-cence, and infection, as well as peripheral nerve injury due to surgical positioning. Further, these patients can develop postdural puncture headache (PDPH) if a dural puncture has occurred during the placement of neuraxial anesthesia. Previously, it was believed that obesity provided a protective mechanism with respect to developing a PDPH after accidental dural puncture. Newer evidence does not support this. The latest evidence suggests mode of delivery to be the largest predictor of development of a PDPH after accidental dural puncture. Parturients who delivered via CS after dural puncture were much less likely to develop a PDPH.[11]

GENERAL ANESTHESIA

General anesthesia for the obese parturient should be avoided whenever possible in order to avoid two major causes of morbidity and mortality, failed intubation and aspiration. Unfortunately these patients are at a high risk of failure of regional anesthesia thus increasing the chances of requiring general anesthesia. Obese patients are at higher risk of developing hypoxemia, hypotension, and aspiration. The risk of failed tracheal intubation is also higher, which is 1 in 280 in the general obstetric population compared to 1 in 2230 in the general surgical population.[12] A 6-year review of obstetric cases of failed intubation in the United Kingdom revealed 36 cases of failed intubation occurring in 8970 obstetric general anesthetics (incidence 1:249).[13] The average BMI of patients with failed intubation was 33.

Preoperative General Anesthesia Considerations

A careful airway examination should be completed immediately prior to induction of general anesthesia, especially in a patient laboring prior to CS, as the airway examination changes during labor. A recent study demonstrated a significant increase in airway Mallampati class pre labor compared to post labor.[14] Thirty-eight of 61 parturients developed a Mallampati class 3 or 4 airway that was independent of duration of labor or fluid administration. As mentioned in the "Difficult Airway" section, a detailed examination should be performed. Otherwise, preparation should be the same, establishing proper IV access and providing aspiration prophylaxis. Again, close proximity of difficult airway equipment is a must.

Intraoperative General Anesthesia Management

Rapid sequence induction is the ideal general anesthetic technique for these patients. Proper positioning of the patient is as important for general anesthesia as it is for regional. As shown in Figure 11-9 above, the patient should be positioned appropriately to improve the laryngoscopic view. Left uterine displacement should be done before inducing anesthesia. Preoxygenation for a full 3 minutes or eight tidal volume breaths over 1 minute with 100% oxygen is recommended. The intubation should be performed via video laryngoscopy, if available. Maintenance utilizing a volatile anesthetic should be done carefully because of the risk of uterine atony. Nitrous oxide can be used as an adjunct to decrease the amount of volatile anesthetic required. Opioid analgesics are administered after delivery. The dosage should be adjusted in obese patients as opioid medication can cause hypoventilation after extubation. Careful monitoring of fluid administration, uterine tone and blood loss should be performed. The morbidly obese patient should be extubated after complete reversal of the muscle relaxant and once the patient is fully awake. During extubation, the risks of airway obstruction, hypoventilation, and aspiration should be kept in mind.

Postoperative General Anesthesia Management

Although the induction and intubation period is a critical time for a morbidly obese parturient, studies have shown that extubation, emergence, and recovery are even more critical.[15] Postoperative pain management is very important in these patients as effective pain control can help with early ambulation and hasten recovery. A multi-modal analgesia approach as discussed above should be adopted to reduce the total amount of opioid consumption. Newer studies have shown regional nerve blocks such as the transversus abdominis plane (TAP) block can be very effective during the first 24 hours after CS. These blocks can be completed in the OR or PACU. Studies have shown that ultrasound-guided TAP blocks reduce analgesic requirements in the first 24 hours after CS.[16] Use of liposomal bupivacaine, a longer acting formulation that slowly releases at the site of injection over time, is currently under investigation for use in TAP blocks for cesarean delivery patients. In the future, this could provide extended pain control and further decrease the amount of opioid pain medications required postoperatively. Adequate pain control, respiratory status, and hemodynamic monitoring are the primary concerns during the immediate recovery period.

COMPLICATIONS OF HIGH-ORDER REPEAT CESAREAN SECTION

There are more than 1,000,000 cesarean sections done per year in the United States, and this accounts for 33% of births in the United States. According to the Centers for Disease Control and Prevention (CDC) National Center for Health Statistics, 87.6% of these patients receive a repeat cesarean section, increasing the risk of placenta accreta. Although planned cesarean section is equal to planned vaginal delivery in terms of mortality, the morbidity is significantly higher than in vaginal delivery.

Cesarean sections in women with five or more previous cesarean sections additionally complicate anesthetic planning. The main risks of high-order repeat cesarean sections include prolonged surgical time secondary to adhesions, placenta previa, placenta accreta, and peripartum hysterectomy. A study from the Shaare Zedek Medical Center in Jerusalem of 108 patients with 6 +/− 1 previous cesarean sections concluded that spinal anesthesia was sufficient for 80 patients (74%) when surgery was performed by an experienced obstetrician.[17] A preoperative ultrasound to look for abnormal placentation including placenta previa and placenta accreta should be performed. If the scan is negative, neuraxial anesthesia should be sufficient for the majority of cases. However, the anesthesiologist should be prepared to change anesthetic management should hemorrhage occur.

The biggest anesthetic concerns are duration of an anesthetic as well as adequate IV access. A CSE is generally placed to afford additional operative time should the surgical team encounter dense adhesions. These patients require at least two large-bore IV lines to enable adequate volume resuscitation, should hemorrhage occur.

Anesthesia in Placenta Accreta Spectrum

Another difficult cesarean section from an anesthesia standpoint involves the placenta accreta spectrum (PAS) disorders, including placenta increta and percreta. Prior to 1972, the risk of PAS was 1 in 7000 pregnancies.[18] The current risk over the last decade is 3 in 1000.[19] Risk for placenta accreta significantly increases with placenta previa, and risk increases greatly with an increasing number of previous cesarean deliveries. The dramatic increase in PAS likely stems from the increased cesarean delivery rate. The major complication of PAS disorders is bleeding, especially with placenta percreta. While the overall mean blood loss for all patients in a study cited by Riveros-Perez was 1500 mL, the median loss for patients with PAS disorders was 2500 mL. Patients with placenta percreta lost significantly more blood, 3250 mL.[20]

Due to the significantly increased risk, early diagnosis is critical. PAS disorders are usually diagnosed with ultrasound first; however, the absence of ultrasound findings does not preclude a PAS diagnosis. MRI is not recommended for initial evaluation of possible PAS, though the American College of Obstetricians and Gynecologists (ACOG) did find improved sensitivity and specificity, as shown in Table 11-4, in detecting PAS with MRI.[21]

The traditional treatment for PAS is cesarean hysterectomy before the onset of labor at approximately 34 weeks. With the advancement of interventional radiology (IR), new techniques were developed with hope of decreasing blood loss and preserving fertility. Due to lack of evidence in favor of IR techniques, planned cesarean hysterectomy remains the treatment of choice at this time. IR techniques are utilized on a case-by-case basis but are considered investigational currently. Uterine artery embolization can be utilized for women who desire to maintain their fertility, but these women need to be counseled on the current lack of evidence supporting this treatment plan.

When the diagnosis of PAS is made early in pregnancy, preparation can be made for a scheduled elective cesarean section with early communication with the blood bank and possible arterial embolization by interventional radiology. When the diagnosis of PAS is made intraoperatively, the placenta can be left in place followed by selective uterine artery embolization with or without concurrent methotrexate.[22] ACOG states that interventional radiology may be useful and IR is especially helpful in cases where no single source of surgical bleeding can be identified.

The *New England Journal of Medicine* released an article on placenta accreta spectrum from April 2018 that lists guidelines for PAS, including antepartum-targeted ultrasonography for women with risk factors for PAS, preoperative counseling, planned delivery with a contingency plan for emergency delivery, and antenatal glucocorticoids. For intrapartum care, delivery should be at a center with a team experienced in PAS care and with a blood bank capable of massive transfusion. Delivery should be scheduled before labor or bleeding. Proper management includes a planned cesarean hysterectomy leaving the placenta in situ. If intraoperative hemorrhage occurs, aggressive volume expansion, transfusion of blood products, and correction of coagulation are vital.

TABLE 11-4 Comparison of Imaging Modalities With Respective Sensitivity and Specificity for Detecting PAS

Type of Imaging	Sensitivity	Specificity	Comments
Ultrasound[20]	77%-93%	71%-96%	Used for initial evaluation, faster, less cost
MRI[21]	94%	84%	May be more appropriate to assess posterior placenta previa and depth of invasion with a suspected placenta percreta, for a patient desiring future fertility

Antepartum Consultation in Placenta Accreta Spectrum

A multidisciplinary team approach is very important in the management of these patients. Anesthesia should be involved as early as possible. The multidisciplinary team may involve the following specialties to optimize the patient's outcome:

- Anesthesiologist
- Obstetrician
- Gynecologic oncologist
- Intensivist
- Maternal-fetal medicine specialist
- Neonatologist
- Urologist
- Hematologist
- Interventional radiologist

According to ACOG guidelines, a guiding principle in management of these patients is to achieve a planned delivery, as data suggest greater blood loss and complications in emergent cesarean hysterectomy versus planned cesarean hysterectomy. Although a planned delivery is the goal, a contingency plan for emergency delivery should be developed for each patient, including an institutional protocol for maternal hemorrhage management. The choices for regional versus general anesthesia should be discussed (Table 11-5). Educating the patient on emergency versus elective delivery is also very important as it would drastically change anesthetic management. Psychosocial support should be offered if required. Conducting a multidisciplinary meeting for these high-risk obstetrical patients allows for preplanning and documentation of the delivery plan.

Preoperative Preparation

Preoperative preparation should first address the safest location for delivery. Is the labor and delivery OR the best option or is the main OR better based on additional personnel and supplies? Does the patient desire IR techniques? If so, a hybrid OR is best as sterility remains intact and radiology services are available. Once the primary plan is in place, an emergency back-up plan needs to be discussed. Patients with placenta accreta may require an emergency preterm delivery because of the sudden onset of massive hemorrhage. Exchange of information and timely communication are essential in the ever-changing environment of these patients' clinical situation. Open communication promotes safe passage of mother and fetus from antepartum to postpartum period.

TABLE 11-5 Benefits of Regional Anesthesia in Placenta Accreta

Intraoperative Benefits	Postoperative Benefits
• Parents experience birth of the baby • Decreased blood loss • Reduced rate of thromboembolic events • Avoidance of endotracheal intubation	• Better pain control than intravenous opioids • Earlier recovery of bowel function • Better ventilation resulting from better pain control • Better participation in physical therapy • Anti-inflammatory effects

Choices of anesthesia:

1. Neuraxial anesthesia: epidural or combined spinal epidural
2. General anesthesia
3. Combination—neuraxial for delivery, general for hysterectomy

A prebriefing before the start of the case is necessary to confirm the plan and make certain that all questions have been answered. This ensures that all team members are present and/or available and are on the same page regarding management.

In order to manage potential massive blood loss, patients with placenta accreta should have at least two large-bore intravenous lines as well as a type and crossmatch for blood products. If peripheral IV access is inadequate, a midline catheter can be placed. If a midline is not possible, a central venous catheter should be placed prior to incision. An arterial line placed prior to incision is recommended; not only for beat-to-beat blood pressure monitoring but also for frequent lab draws that may become necessary as the case progresses. Communication with the blood bank is especially important, and author Denis Snegovskikh, M.D., at Yale University School of Medicine reports his institution requests blood products as shown in Table 11-6 depending on whether the case is routine or complicated.[22] During the surgery, frequent check-ins with the surgeons should be done for better coordination and anticipation of potential blood loss. If a cesarean hysterectomy for abnormal placentation is needed, a multicenter review reported an average blood loss of 2526 mL and an average of 6.6 U PRBCs transfused.[23] Crossmatched blood products need to be in the room and checked prior to incision.

Intraoperative Management

As discussed in the preoperative section, several types of anesthesia are appropriate for management of known placenta accreta patients undergoing cesarean hysterectomy.

1. Epidural. Knowing the epidural catheter is functioning prior to incision is the greatest strength of this technique as almost all cesarean hysterectomy cases will last beyond the duration of a spinal anesthetic. The main drawback is the potential for a less dense block or a "patchy" block which may require conversion to general anesthesia prior to delivery.
2. CSE is a second option where the patient receives the dense spinal block but also has an epidural catheter placed which can be dosed as the spinal recedes. With a CSE, there is no guarantee the catheter will be functional when redosing becomes necessary.
3. A third option is placing a spinal or CSE with the intent of the patient remaining awake until delivery and then transitioning to general anesthesia for the remainder of the procedure.
4. The final option is conducting the entire case under general anesthesia from start to finish.

TABLE 11-6 Recommended Blood Products to be Available for Cesarean Section for PAS Cases[22]

Type of PAS case	RBCs	FFP	Platelets	Cryoprecipitate
Routine	4 U	4 U		
Complicated	10 U	10 U	10 U	10 U

Complications during cases of placenta accreta, in addition to massive hemorrhage, include conversion from regional anesthesia to general anesthesia, cesarean hysterectomy, and disseminated intravascular coagulation (DIC). In many cases of placenta accreta, neuraxial anesthesia may be appropriate, as it does not contribute to increased maternal morbidity and reduces the amount of blood loss.[24] The choice of neuraxial versus general anesthesia depends on the patient's airway, the presence of any coagulopathy, the anticipated blood loss, the duration of the surgery, the possibility of large fluid shifts, and the ability of the patient to tolerate sympathectomy and decreased preload and afterload of neuraxial anesthesia.

To handle the large fluid shifts and hemodynamic changes of PAS patients during cesarean section, Riveros-Perez et al. at the University of Colorado Hospital recommend CSE anesthesia until umbilical cord clamping and general anesthesia after cord clamping. They recommend the technique of CSE converted to general anesthesia in order to safely access the airway early. Intraoperatively, Snegovskikh et al. recommend that laboratory studies (prothrombin time [PT], partial thromboplastin time [PTT], platelet count, fibrinogen level) are drawn hourly if the massive transfusion protocol requires activation.

The anesthesiologist must be prepared to initiate massive blood product resuscitation at any moment. A rapid infuser, such as the Belmont pictured in Figure 11-13, can greatly assist should hemorrhage occur. The Belmont can infuse up to 1000 mL/min, which can equal the rate of blood loss on the operative field. Having plenty of help in the operating room is essential during these times.

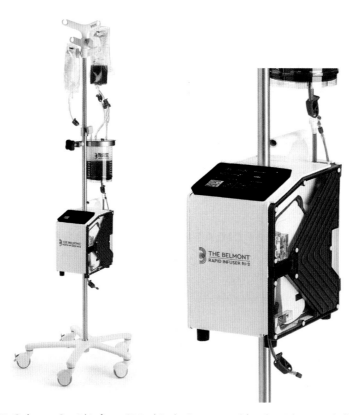

FIGURE 11-13 Belmont Rapid Infuser RI-2, this device warms blood products and allows infusions ranging from 2.5 to 1000 mL/min (Belmont Medical Technologies, Billerica, MA).

Blood conservation techniques such as the use of tranexamic acid and autologous cell salvage can help minimize allogeneic red blood cell transfusion to patients at high risk of massive obstetric hemorrhage. Parturients with low preoperative hemoglobin concentrations, rare blood types (eg, Bombay), and/or those who refuse transfusion products including Jehovah's witnesses can all benefit. Cell salvage is a technique where surgical field blood loss is collected and washed. The red cells are then returned to the patient. Previously, cell salvage has been underutilized in obstetric surgery for fear of causing amniotic fluid embolism (AFE), infection, or DIC. Though large, randomized, prospective studies are lacking, retrospective studies have failed to demonstrate any increase in the incidence of AFE, infection, or DIC when cell salvage is used during CS. Though not necessary for routine cesarean deliveries, cell salvage should be considered for PAS disorder deliveries.[23]

Postoperative Management

The CSE anesthesia technique not only helps with safe delivery of the baby and participation of the mother; it can be used effectively for postoperative pain management. Postoperative epidural infusion can help reduce the overall opioid consumption and provide effective pain control for the patient. A repeat coagulation profile should be reviewed prior to removal of the epidural catheter.

Postoperative management also depends on whether any of the complications listed below occur intraoperatively. Quantitative blood loss compared to the calculated maximal allowable blood loss, as well as clinical assessment of patient hemodynamics, will assist with the decision to transfuse blood products. A complete blood count (CBC), coagulation studies such as a prothrombin time/international normalized ratio (PT/INR), activated partial thromboplastin time (aPTT), and fibrinogen level can further assist with transfusion decision-making. Point-of-care thromboelastography (TEG) demonstrates patient's clotting in real time and can be invaluable with regards to product replacement. A decision must also be made on whether postoperative care should be in the postanesthesia care unit or the intensive care unit.

ANESTHESIA COMPLICATIONS IN CESAREAN SECTION OF A PATIENT WITH PLACENTA ACCRETA SPECTRUM

- Massive obstetric hemorrhage
- Disseminated intravascular coagulopathy
- Hysterectomy; surgical injury to the ureters, bladder, bowel, or neurovascular structures
- Adult respiratory distress syndrome
- Acute transfusion reaction
- Electrolyte imbalance
- Renal failure

REFERENCES

1. Palmer CM, D'Angelo R, Paech MJ. *Handbook of Obstetric Anesthesia*. Trowbridge, UK: Cromwell Press; 2002.
2. Centers for Disease Control and Prevention. Adult Obesity Facts. February 6, 2019. Available at https://www.cdc.gov/obesity/data/adult.html.
3. Centers for Disease Control and Prevention. Prepregnancy Body Mass Index by Maternal Characteristics and State: Data From the Birth Certificate, 2014. February 6, 2019. Available at https://www.cdc.gov/nchs/data/nvsr/nvsr65/nvsr65_06.pdf.
4. Tyner J, Rayburn W. Emergency cesarean delivery. *Obstet Gynecol Clin North Am*. 2013;40:37-45.
5. Hughes SC, Levinson G, Rosen MA, Shnider SN. *Shnider and Levinson's Anesthesia for Obstetrics*. Philadelphia: Lippincott Williams & Wilkins; 2002.
6. Anderson NR. When to use a midline catheter. *Nursing*. 2005;35(4):68.
7. Carvalho B. Respiratory depression after neuraxial opioids in the obstetric setting. *Anesth Analg*. 2008;107(3):956-961.
8. Lee AJ, Smiley RM. Phenylephrine infusions during cesarean section under spinal anesthesia. *Int Anesthesiol Clin*. 2014;52(2):29-47.
9. Hodgkinson R, Husain FJ. Caesarean section associated with gross obesity. *Br J Anaesth*. 1980;52(9):919-923.
10. Perlow JH, Morgan MA. Massive maternal obesity and perioperative Cesarean morbidity. *Am J Obstet Gynecol*. 1994;170:560-565.
11. Gaiser R. Anesthetic considerations in the obese parturient. *Clin Obstet Gynecol*. 2016;59(1):193-203.
12. Samsoon GL, Young JR. Difficult tracheal intubation: a retrospective study. *Anaesthesia*. 1987;42:487-490.
13. Barnardo PD, Jenkins JG. Failed tracheal intubation in obstetrics: a 6-year review in a UK region. *Anaesthesia*. 2000;55:690-694.
14. Kodali BS, Chandrasekhar S, Bulich LN, Topulos GP, Datta S. Airway changes during labor and delivery. *Anesthesiology*. 2008;108:357-362.
15. Mhyre JM, Riesner MN, Polley LS, Naughton NN. A series of anesthesia-related maternal deaths in Michigan. *Anesthesiology*. 2007;106(6):1096-1104.
16. Mankikar MG, Sardesai SP, Ghodki PS. Ultrasound-guided transversus abdominis plane block for post-operative analgesia in patients undergoing caesarean section. *Indian J Anaesth*. 2016;60(4):253-257.
17. Ioscovich A, Mirochnitchenko E, Halpern S, et al. Perioperative anaesthetic management of high-order repeat caesarean section: audit of practice in a university-affiliated medical centre. *Int J Obstet Anesth*. 2009;18:314-319.
18. Breen JL, Neubecker R, Gregori CA, et al. Placenta accreta, increta, and percreta. A survey of 40 cases. *Obstet Gynecol*. 1977;49(1):43-47.
19. Belfort MA. Placenta accreta. *Am J Obstet Gynecol*. 2008;203(5):430-439.
20. Riveros-Perez E, Wood C. Retrospective analysis of obstetric and anesthetic management of patients with placenta accreta spectrum disorders. *Int J Gynaecol Obstet*. 2018;140:370-374.
21. American College of Obstetricians and Gynecologists. Obstetric Care Consensus. February 7, 2019. Available at https://www.acog.org/Clinical-Guidance-and-Publications/Obstetric-Care-Consensus-Series/Placenta-Accreta-Spectrum.
22. Snegovskikh D, Clebone A, Norwitz E. Anesthetic management of patients with placenta accreta and resuscitation strategies for associated massive hemorrhage. *Curr Opin Anaesthesiol*. 2011;24:274-281.
23. Allam J, Cox M, Yentis SM. Cell salvage in obstetrics. *Int J Obstet Anesth*. 2008;17(1):37-45.
24. Chestnut DH, Dewan DM, Redick LF, et al. Anesthetic management for obstetric hysterectomy: a multi-institutional study. *Anesthesiology*. 1989;70:607-610.

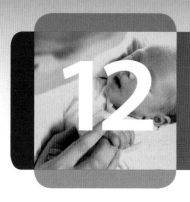

12

The Role of Interventional Radiology in the Management of the Difficult Cesarean Delivery

Joanna Kee-Sampson, Travis E. Meyer, Daniel Siragusa

INTRODUCTION AND HISTORICAL PERSPECTIVES

Endovascular interventions performed by interventional radiologists for high-risk obstetric cases can decrease morbidity and mortality in the peripartum period. In the interest of best maternal outcomes, the management of high-risk pregnancies should include interventional radiology as a key member of the multidisciplinary team.

The father of modern interventional radiology, Charles Dotter, published a seminal article in 1963 describing the recanalization of an artery through a small hole in the artery,[1] without the need to perform surgery. With refinement in transarterial techniques and advances in equipment over the years, the scope of interventional radiologists has expanded to include an increasing range of procedures for an ever-widening range of indications.[2] Transarterial techniques are particularly suited to halt or prevent bleeding in any organ system because they are minimally invasive and highly effective. The first case of transcatheter embolization for an obstetric indication was published in 1979,[3] describing the case of a 22-year-old with massive postpartum hemorrhage after vaginal delivery which was inadequately controlled by packing, hysterectomy, and bilateral internal iliac artery ligation. Embolization of the left internal pudendal artery was eventually performed by an interventional radiologist, which succeeded at stabilizing the patient.

Transarterial techniques are now used for a number of obstetric and gynecologic indications including abnormal placentation, menorrhagia, and postpartum hemorrhage or postpartum bleeding.[4] In this chapter, we will describe the obstetric indications for transarterial therapy and include a discussion on the infrastructure and set-up for the treatment, management, and predelivery planning of high-risk pregnancies by the obstetrics-interventional radiology team.

PREDISPOSING CONDITIONS TO PERIPARTUM HEMORRHAGE

Placenta Accreta Spectrum

The decidua basalis layer of the placenta prevents abnormal adherence of the placenta to the myometrium and enables placental separation during labor. Placenta accreta, morbidly adherent placenta, and abnormal placental implantation are terminologies that were used in reference to the abnormal adherence of the placenta to the myometrium from ingrowth of the chorionic villi through the decidua basalis. *Placenta accreta spectrum* is the updated terminology for this pathology. The depth of chorionic villi invasion characterizes the severity of the placental abnormality and is classically described as placenta accreta, increta, and percreta denoting chorionic invasion not invading, partially invading, and full-thickness invasion of the myometrium beyond the serosa. In placenta percreta, the abnormal placenta may adhere to the surrounding abdominopelvic organs and musculature. After delivery, when the abnormal placenta does not separate from the uterus, postpartum hemorrhage may occur, potentially leading to hemorrhagic shock, coagulopathy, hysterectomy, and death.[5] Women with placenta accreta spectrum on average lose 3 to 5 L of blood at delivery, and 40% require transfusion of more than 10 units of packed red blood cells. Maternal mortality has been reported at 7%.[6,7]

Incidence and Risk Factors for Placenta Accreta Spectrum

The incidence of placenta accreta spectrum has progressively increased from 1:4027 pregnancies in the 1970s to 1:533 pregnancies from 1982-2002, to 1:272 pregnancies in 2016.[8,9] This dramatic increase has mainly been attributed to the increase in the rates of cesarean section, which now exceeds 30% in developed countries.[5,10] Furthermore, the incidence of placenta accreta spectrum increases with the incidence of placenta previa, which has also been strongly correlated with a history of prior cesarean section. In any individual woman, the larger the number of previous cesarean sections, the greater the risk of abnormal placental implantation, increasing from a risk of 3.3% in a woman without prior cesarean sections to 67% in those with four or more prior cesarean sections.[5,8] Other minor risk factors that predispose to the development of placenta accreta spectrum are advanced maternal age, multiparity, prior uterine surgery, and endometrial curettage.

Diagnosis of Placenta Accreta Spectrum

Ultrasound

Screening for placenta accreta spectrum occurs at the routine 18 to 20 week ultrasound examination, with extra care at imaging the anterior myometrium and bladder should the patient have any relevant history that would increase the risk of developing placenta accreta spectrum.[11] The reported sensitivity and specificity of sonography in the diagnosis of placenta accreta spectrum were 91% and 97%, respectively, in a systematic review and meta-analysis.[12] The absence of relevant sonographic findings, however, should not preclude a diagnosis of placenta accreta spectrum as clinical risk factors are equally important predictors.[8]

The normal sonographic appearance of the placenta-myometrium junction should show a thin hypoechoic line separating the placenta from the inner myometrium. The subplacental blood flow pattern should be organized and parallel the myometrium.[11] As previously discussed, placenta previa is a risk factor for developing placenta accreta spectrum. When placenta previa is seen on ultrasound examination, careful additional imaging with color Doppler and transvaginal probes should be performed to exclude concurrent placenta accreta. Other abnormal findings seen in placenta accreta spectrum are placental lacunae, increased vascularity around the uterus, irregular bladder wall, absence of the retroplacental clear space, and anterior myometrial thickness less than 1 mm.[11,13]

Magnetic Resonance Imaging

Magnetic resonance imaging (MRI) is indicated when there are risk factors for placenta accreta spectrum but ultrasound findings are equivocal, when there is a posterior placenta previa, or to assess the depth of myometrial invasion in percreta.[8,11,13] MRI is also a useful adjunctive imaging tool in the preoperative planning of cesarean section delivery and peripartum hysterectomy.[13] The sensitivity and specificity of MRI in the diagnosis of placenta accreta spectrum are comparable to sonography; however, it is more expensive, not as widely available, and requires more expertise for interpretation, and therefore, it is not recommended as a first-line imaging modality for placenta accreta spectrum.[8]

MRI findings seen in an invasive placenta are uterine bulging, heterogeneity of the placenta with increased vascularity, and dark bands in the placenta extending from the myometrium, and in later pregnancy, focal myometrial interruptions may be seen (Figure 12-1). In placenta percreta, the placenta may invade the surrounding organs and structures.[11] The administration of gadolinium-based contrast may improve the delineation of the placenta-myometrium junction; however, its use during pregnancy is controversial because of its ability to cross the placenta and circulate in the amniotic fluid. The effects of gadolinium on the fetus are unknown. The American College of Radiology Manual on Contrast Media recommends that gadolinium-based contrast medium should be administered with caution to pregnant women and only when the potential significant benefits outweigh the possible but unknown risks to the fetus.[14]

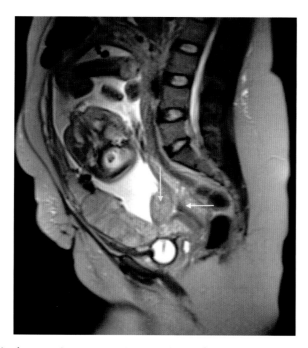

FIGURE 12-1 Sagittal magnetic resonance imaging (MRI) of a 32-year-old woman with placenta previa and accreta. The placenta (yellow arrow) is covering the cervical os (white arrow). There is also loss of the normal uterus-placental hypointense zone, consistent with placenta accreta.

Uterine Atony

Uterine atony is the failure of the uterus to contract after delivery. It is the most common cause of peripartum hemorrhage.[15] Uterotonic agents should be the first treatment for abnormal postpartum hemorrhage due to uterine atony according to the American College of Obstetricians and Gynecologists (ACOG) guidelines, based on good and consistent scientific evidence (level A).[16] When manual uterine massage and uterotonic medications fail to adequately control the blood loss, prompt surgical or transarterial intervention is warranted.

Although hysterectomy remains the most definitive solution, it is also more invasive than alternatives and of course removes the option for future pregnancies. Uterine or internal iliac artery ligation via laparoscopic approaches can minimize recovery times but are also considered more invasive than transarterial embolization. Bilateral internal iliac artery ligation has success rates of 40% to 100%, while bilateral uterine artery ligation has success rates of approximately 92%.[17] Transarterial embolization of the uterine arteries has reported success rates of approximately 85% to 100%.[18-20] In locations where interventional radiology is not readily available, laparoscopic ligation is an important option. In cases where embolization fails, laparoscopy may be pursued before complete hysterectomy; however, if ligation has been performed first, then embolization can be very technically difficult with lower success rates leaving hysterectomy as the only remaining option.[21]

Genital Lacerations

Perineal and genital tract lacerations can occur in up to 80% of deliveries.[22] Common sites for laceration include the perineum and vagina but can also occur on the labia, clitoris, urethra, and cervix. The severity of lacerations varies from minor lacerations that affect the skin or superficial structures of the perineum to more severe lacerations that damage the muscles of the anal sphincter complex and rectum. Risk factors for more severe lacerations include induced labor, epidural anesthesia, increased birth weight of the infant, and operative or augmented vaginal delivery.[23]

For mild lacerations, no intervention is usually required. For moderate lacerations, approximation of the tissue with absorbable suture and packing of the vagina is often sufficient.[24] In cases of significant hemorrhage or where suturing does not control blood loss, interventional or operative management is the next step.

Postpartum genital tract lacerations often involve the vaginal artery which is a branch of the anterior division of the internal iliac artery. Selective embolization with Gelfoam or coils can provide excellent control of the hemorrhage.[25] As with all pelvic embolizations, a postembolization pelvic angiogram at the level of L3-L4 is warranted to exclude alternative sources of bleeding not previously identified before removing arterial access.[26] In cases where active extravasation is not identified, empiric embolization of the bilateral uterine arteries can be performed depending on the location of the laceration. Temporary embolization of the internal iliac artery on the side of the laceration is acceptable if arterial ligation or hysterectomy is the only competing alternative in the setting of unidentified hemorrhage.

DELIVERY PLANNING AND DELIVERY

Facility and Multidisciplinary Team

Because of the risk of massive peripartum hemorrhage and associated morbidities, the American College of Obstetricians and Gynecologists strongly recommends (grade 1B) that perinatal care in a patient with placenta accreta spectrum should take place in a facility capable of level III or IV maternal care where there is adequate blood bank, personnel, and medical subspecialty support and experience.[8] The availability of a multidisciplinary team consisting of in-house obstetrician gynecologists, gynecologic oncologists, anesthesiologists, other surgical subspecialties, and immediate availability of interventional radiologists are essential to providing the best maternal outcomes. In a retrospective cohort study of deliveries complicated by placenta accreta spectrum, women who delivered in a medical center with a multidisciplinary care team had a greater than 50% risk reduction of early morbidity compared with those who delivered in a less equipped medical center.[27]

Planned Versus Emergency Cesarean Hysterectomy

Generally, a planned cesarean delivery is preferred over an emergency cesarean hysterectomy as this leads to better outcomes.[5,8] The timing of planned delivery should be tailored to each patient's circumstance, taking into consideration clinical stability and the degree of placental invasion. Some authors prefer to deliver at 34 weeks for the best maternal and fetal outcomes.[5,28] The ACOG recommends scheduled delivery between 34 0/7 to 35 6/7 weeks of gestation in a stable patient.[8] The standard of care is cesarean hysterectomy at the time of delivery, but newer, uterus-conserving techniques have been described to preserve fertility in select patients.[5,8]

The interventional radiology team is typically notified ahead of the planned delivery date so that adequate staff and physicians are made available.

When concurrent radiological interventions are considered, delivery should occur in a hybrid operating suite whenever possible. The hybrid operating suite offers several advantages over the traditional operating room; it has the room to accommodate additional medical personnel and equipment and offers advanced imaging capabilities of a better quality than portable C-arm fluoroscopy, while maintaining the sterility standards and lighting of a traditional operating room (Figure 12-2). Additionally, the logistics, difficulties, and potential complications in the transportation of an unstable patient between the operating room and interventional radiology suite are avoided.[29]

Contingency plans should be in place in the event of an emergency, whether it may be an emergent delivery in a patient with placenta accreta or massive postpartum hemorrhage from other etiologies. Although interventional radiologists are not usually in-house outside of regular daytime hours, in tertiary medical centers, they are available on call around the clock should the need for emergent endovascular procedures arise. There are no published guidelines that specifically address the expected on-call response time for interventional radiology teams for emergent obstetric cases. In treating similarly acute and critically ill trauma patients in a level I/II trauma center, the American College of Surgeons require interventional radiologists to be available within 30 minutes to perform complex imaging studies or interventional procedures.[30]

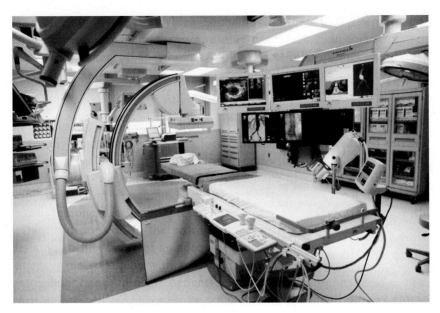

FIGURE 12-2 Hybrid operating suite. (Reprinted with permission from Franco KL, Thourani VH. *Cardiothoracic Surgery Review*. Philadelphia: Wolters Kluwer; 2012.)

ENDOVASCULAR INTERVENTIONS

Endovascular interventions for intrapartum or postpartum hemorrhage can be divided into two general categories: temporary occlusion and embolization. Temporary occlusion can either occur at the infrarenal aortic level, common iliac arteries, or at the level of the internal iliac arteries. Embolization can be achieved by using various embolic agents and may need to include arteries in addition to the uterine artery, such as the internal pudendal artery. Although the first case of transcatheter embolization for an obstetric indication was published in 1979 detailing the embolization of the internal pudendal artery to achieve hemostasis,[3] it was not until 1997 that prophylactic perioperative internal iliac artery balloon occlusion in cases of abnormal placental invasion was first reported.[31] Preference is to occlude or embolize as selectively as feasible given the urgency of the intervention. Initial preparation is key to fast and effective hemostasis. Ensure that your team has a variety of balloon sizes and embolic agents available to accommodate any anticipated findings during the procedure.

Embolization

Embolization is usually fast and effective in controlling unmitigated hemorrhage.[32] The absence of positive findings of active hemorrhage on angiography should not prevent or delay the embolization of the bilateral uterine arteries.[33] Additional arterial embolization, including but not limited to the internal pudendal or entire internal iliac arteries may be required (Figure 12-3A-D).

Choice of Embolic Agents

The choice of embolic agents depends on angiographic findings, operator preference, final catheter position, and the desired duration of stasis. Gelfoam (Pfizer, New York,

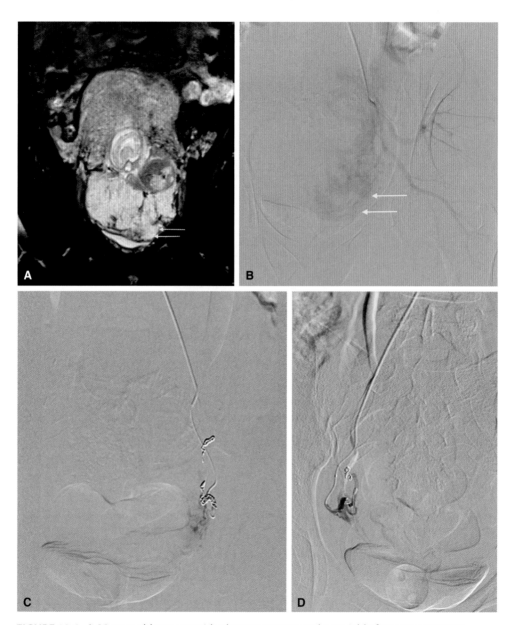

FIGURE 12-3 A 28-year-old woman with placenta accreta and nonviable fetus presenting to interventional radiology for preoperative embolization. (A) Magnetic resonance imaging (MRI) shows loss of the normal uterus-placental hypointense zone and bulging of the placenta toward the dome of the urinary bladder (arrows). (B) Left internal iliac angiogram shows corresponding enhancement of the uterus and placenta (arrows). (C and D) Embolization of the bilateral uterine arteries was performed with particles and coils, with cessation of blood flow to the uterus after embolization.

USA) can be cut into pledgets or macerated into a slurry with dilute contrast (Figure 12-4). In most cases, it is resorbed with recanalization of the vessel in 4 to 6 weeks.[34] Permanent embolic agents can be divided into three main categories: liquids (N-butyl cyanoacrylate), particulates (polyvinyl alcohol particles or spherical particles), or coils/vascular plugs

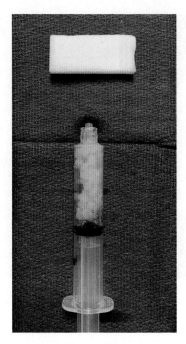

FIGURE 12-4 Gelfoam slurry.

(Figure 12-5). Although coil or plug embolization has the benefit of quick deployment, it often requires more distal catheterization prior to embolization than is necessary with particles or Gelfoam as rich vascular collateralization of the pelvis can cause failure of proximal embolization alone.

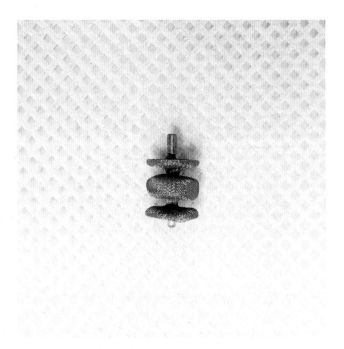

FIGURE 12-5 Vascular plug.

Interventional Radiology in Embolization

Transarterial procedures usually begin with access via the common femoral artery using the modified Seldinger technique with ultrasound guidance or by fluoroscopy and palpation. Less commonly, procedures can be performed from an upper extremity arterial access (brachial or radial). Ultrasound guidance is particularly helpful in women with small-diameter femoral arteries or diminished pulses secondary to hypovolemia. A single puncture of the common femoral artery allows catheterization of both the pelvic arteries using a Waltman loop[35] or dedicated uterine artery catheter. Given the time and effort required to form the Waltman loop, many angiographers will begin investigation and treatment of the side contralateral to the access point. In situations where time is critical, communication from the obstetric team about findings during delivery or intraoperatively which may indicate the side of the hemorrhage is important. Often interventional radiology suites or hybrid operating rooms are set up for right femoral artery access and given no benefit to one side versus the other in the absence of further knowledge about the exact location of the hemorrhage, any delay that would be caused by changing the room setup should be avoided.

Modified Seldinger Technique

- The modified Seldinger technique sequence starts with a puncture of the anterior arterial wall with a 21-gauge needle, followed by threading a guidewire through the needle into the arterial lumen. Subsequently, over the guidewire, a sheath is placed into the artery to maintain access. The sideport of the sheath should be flushed with saline.
- If prolonged vascular access is anticipated, a pressurized flush bag of heparinized saline may be attached to the sideport. A catheter can then be advanced to the contralateral common iliac artery.
- Usually, the contralateral anterior oblique view (approximately 30°) is recommended in order to delineate the location of the anterior division of the internal iliac artery.
- A hemipelvic angiogram from the common or internal iliac artery is helpful to locate the origin and course of the uterine artery as well as identify any additional vessels with active extravasation.
- Direct catheterization of the uterine artery with a 5 French catheter is often easily accomplished as the vessel is almost always hypertrophied from the gravid state.
- If hypovolemia has caused vasoconstriction limiting access to the uterine artery, then a microcatheter and microwire combination should be advanced into the uterine artery.
- Additionally, more distal catheter placement with a microcatheter may be desired if a contrast blush is readily identified and achieving closer proximity will not delay embolization.
- Gelfoam slurry or particulate embolization can be performed to stasis. Coil or plug embolization of the proximal uterine artery is rarely required.
- Postembolization angiogram after withdrawal of the 5 French catheter back into the internal iliac artery is necessary as the altered blood flow and pressure dynamics from embolization may allow visualization of previously occult site of vascular injury.
- If intraoperative hemorrhage control is not achieved with uterine artery embolization, hemipelvic embolization of the internal iliac artery can be performed without concern.[36]

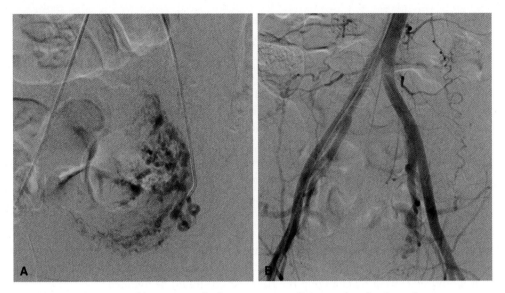

FIGURE 12-6 A 20-year-old woman with placenta accreta discovered at the time of cesarean section presenting to interventional radiology for uterine artery embolization prior to hysterectomy. (A) Left uterine arteriogram demonstrates the typical hypertrophied appearance of the artery in a gravid state. (B) A "pruned" appearance of the bilateral uterine arteries after embolization.

- After the contralateral side has been evaluated and embolized, the catheter can be directed to the ipsilateral iliac vasculature by formation of a Waltman loop or by use of catheters designed for this purpose. Again, angulation of the portable C-arm fluoroscope or image intensifier to 30° contralateral anterior oblique view is helpful.
- Catheterization, angiographic evaluation, and embolization of the ipsilateral side are identical to the prior steps taken for the contralateral side.
- After embolization of both uterine arteries and any additional vasculature needed to obtain hemostasis, a general pelvic angiogram from a posterior-anterior angulation is helpful to exclude any prominent collateral supply which may cause secondary rebleeding or embolization failure (Figure 12-6A and B).
- Although arteriotomy closure devices are commonly used in routine outpatient procedures, careful consideration should be exercised when used in patients with hypovolemia as small artery diameters can increase the risk for complications.[37,38]

Risks and Complications From Embolization

The risk of major complications from bilateral uterine artery or pelvic artery embolization increases with the contiguous vascular territory embolized; however, the incidence of necrosis, venous thrombosis, or peripheral neuropathy remains acceptably low.[39] Additionally, the risk of complications in future pregnancies is not above the general population.[40]

Balloon Occlusion

Prophylactic or intraoperative balloon occlusion to decrease intraoperative blood loss has been reported extensively in the literature, with mixed conclusions. Some authors report statistically significant decrease in intraoperative blood loss with balloon occlusion usage,[41-46] while others report no therapeutic advantage of balloon occlusion.[47-50]

Most of the published studies constitute level 3 evidence. To date, there have not been any large, randomized control trials that have been published evaluating the efficacy of balloon occlusion.

Internal Iliac Balloon Occlusion

Prophylactic perioperative internal iliac artery balloon occlusion (IIBO) in cases of abnormal placental invasion was first reported in 1997.[31] Since then, bilateral internal iliac balloon placement has become more common as a precautionary measure for expected high blood loss deliveries and cesarean sections.

- If a hybrid operating suite is not available, the procedure can be performed in advance of a planned surgery in the interventional radiology suite with local anesthesia or moderate sedation and the patient then transferred to the obstetrical surgical suite. Alternatively, the procedure can be performed with portable C-arm fluoroscopy in the operating room.
- Bilateral femoral arterial access is required as one balloon is placed in the contralateral internal iliac artery via each vascular sheath. A sheath size of 6 French is recommended as the catheter size is often 5 French, but the ultimate sheath size placed does depend on the balloon diameter required. In contrast to balloon catheters used for dilation of atherosclerotic stenosis, the balloons used in internal iliac artery occlusion are compliant and the diameter of the balloon corresponds with the volume delivered (Figure 12-7). The larger sheath allows a pressurized flush bag of heparinized saline to be attached to the sideport and titrated to a slow drip or controlled via an IV pump.
- Placement and volume required for adequate balloon occlusion should be performed and confirmed before the planned surgical procedure begins. Additionally, if the patient is to be transferred from the interventional radiology suite to the obstetric operating room, the sheaths and catheters should be sutured in place and reinforced with ample tape. Transfer of the patient via "slider boards" or other assistive devices is preferred to decrease motion and hip flexion thereby decreasing the chances of balloon migration after placement.

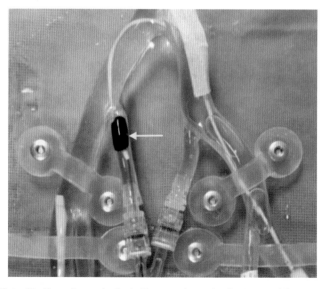

FIGURE 12-7 Inflated balloon (arrow) of a balloon catheter in the internal iliac artery of this model.

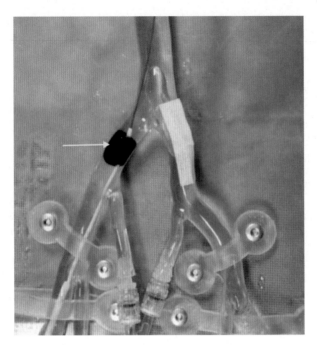

FIGURE 12-8 Inflated balloon (arrow) of a balloon catheter in the common iliac artery of this model.

- Removal of the balloon catheters should be performed as soon as the surgeon deems them no longer clinically needed in order to minimize the risk of arterial thrombosis.
- Vascular sheath removal may be performed after primary closure or after recovery from anesthesia.

Infrarenal Aortic Balloon Occlusion

Depending on the vascular collateralization of the pelvis or the extent of abnormal placental invasion to surrounding structures, adequate hemostatic control may not be achieved with occlusion of the bilateral internal iliac arteries alone. Bilateral common iliac or infrarenal aortic occlusion is occasionally needed to complete a hysterectomy (Figure 12-8).

The first use of intra-abdominal aortic balloon occlusion for hemorrhage was in the setting of battle trauma described in 1956 by Hughes.[51] Presently, abdominal aortic balloon occlusion in the setting of expected peripartum hemorrhage is under investigation. Some operators and studies suggest that occlusion should happen before delivery, and others suggest that occlusion be achieved after delivery.[52] A balloon occlusion time of up to 30 minutes is considered safe and adequate time to control bleeding.[52,53] Lower extremity arterial thrombosis is the most notable complication, with rates of 0% to 10% reported in the literature.[46,54-56]

Depending on the availability of supplies, a Resuscitative Endovascular Balloon Occlusion of the Aorta (REBOA) kit may be used from the trauma bay or vascular surgical suite, or the interventional radiology department may use a variety of balloons often used for endovascular aortic aneurysm repair cases. Although technical success is excellent, complications can arise when inflation times are prolonged or technical considerations are not observed.[57]

🛡 SAFEGUARDS

- The timing of planned delivery should be tailored to each patient's circumstance, taking into consideration clinical stability and the degree of placental invasion. Some authors prefer to deliver at 34 weeks for the best maternal and fetal outcomes.[5,28] The ACOG recommends scheduled delivery between 34 0/7 to 35 6/7 weeks of gestation in a stable patient.[8] The standard of care is cesarean hysterectomy at the time of delivery, but newer, uterus-conserving techniques have been described to preserve fertility in select patients.[5,8]

- There are no published guidelines that specifically address the expected on-call response time for interventional radiology teams for emergent obstetric cases. In treating similarly acute and critically ill trauma patients in a level I/II trauma center, the American College of Surgeons require interventional radiologists to be available within 30 minutes to perform complex imaging studies or interventional procedures.[30]

- Preference is to occlude or embolize as selectively as feasible in cases of emergent endovascular intervention for intrapartum or postpartum hemorrhage.

- Often interventional radiology suites or hybrid operating rooms are set up for right femoral artery access. Given that there is no benefit to accessing the right versus the left femoral artery in the absence of knowledge about the exact location of the hemorrhage, any delay that would be caused by changing the room setup should be avoided.

- Although arteriotomy closure devices are commonly used in routine outpatient procedures, careful consideration should be exercised when used in patients with hypovolemia as small artery diameters can increase the risk for complications.[37,38]

REFERENCES

1. Dotter CT, Judkins MP. Transluminal treatment of arteriosclerotic obstruction: description of a new technic and a preliminary report of its application. *Circulation*. 1964;30:654-670.
2. Murphy TP, Soares GM. The evolution of interventional radiology. *Semin Intervent Radiol*. 2005;22(1):6-9.
3. Heaston DK, Mineau DE, Brown BJ, Miller FJ. Transcatheter arterial embolization for control of persistent massive puerperal hemorrhage after bilateral surgical hypogastric artery ligation. *Am J Roentgenol*. 1979;133:152-154.
4. Salazar GMM, Petrozza JC, Walker TG. Transcatheter endovascular techniques for management of obstetrical and gynecologic emergencies. *Tech Vasc Interv Radiol*. 2009;12(2):139-147.
5. Hull AD, Resnik R. Placenta accreta and postpartum hemorrhage. *Clin Obstet Gynecol*. 2010;53(1):228-236.
6. O'Brien JM, Barton JR, Donaldson ES. The management of placenta percreta: conservative and operative strategies. *Am J Obstet Gynecol*. 1996;175(6):1632-1638.
7. Hudon L, Belfort MA, Broome DR. Diagnosis and management of placenta percreta: a review. *Obstet Gynecol Surv*. 1998;53(8):509-517.
8. American College of Obstetricians and Gynecologists. Obstetric care consensus no. 7: placenta accreta spectrum. *Obstet Gynecol*. 2018;132:e259-e275.
9. Wu S, Kocherginsky M, Hibbard JU. Abnormal placentation: twenty-year analysis. *Am J Obstet Gynecol*. 2005;192(5):1458-1461.
10. Martin JA, Hamilton BE, Osterman MJK, Driscoll AK, Drake P. National vital statistics reports. Centers for Disease Control and Prevention, National Center for Health Statistics, National Vital Statistics System. 2018;67(1):1-55.

11. Baughman WC, Corteville JE, Shah RR. Placenta accreta: spectrum of US and MR imaging findings. *Radiographics*. 2008;28:1905-1916.

12. D'Antonio F, Iacovella C, Bhide A. Prenatal identification of invasive placentation using ultrasound: systematic review and meta-analysis. *Ultrasound Obstet Gynecol*. 2013;42:509-517.

13. Kilcoyne A, Shenoy-Bhangle AS, Roberts DJ, Sisodia RC, Gervais DA, Lee SI. MRI of placenta accreta, placenta increta, and placenta percreta: pearls and pitfalls. *Am J Roentgenol*. 2017;208:214-221.

14. *ACR Manual on Contrast Media, Version 10.3*. American College of Radiology; 2018. Available at https://www.acr.org/-/media/ACR/Files/Clinical-Resources/Contrast_Media.pdf. Accessed December 9, 2018.

15. Mousa HA, Blum J, Abou El Senoun G, Shakur H, Alfirevic Z. Treatment for primary postpartum haemorrhage. *Cochrane Database Syst Rev*. 2014;2(2):CD003249.

16. Shields LE, Goffman D, Caughey AB. Postpartum hemorrhage. *Obstet Gynecol*. 2017;130(4):e168-e186.

17. Wee L, Barron J, Toye R. Management of severe postpartum haemorrhage by uterine artery embolization. *Br J Anaesth*. 2004;93(4):591-594.

18. Spreu A, Abgottspon F, Baumann MU, Kettenbach J, Surbek D. Efficacy of pelvic artery embolisation for severe postpartum hemorrhage. *Arch Gynecol Obstet*. 2017;296(6):1117-1124.

19. Aoki M, Tokue H, Miyazaki M, Shibuya K, Hirasawa S, Oshima K. Primary postpartum hemorrhage: outcome of uterine artery embolization. *Br J Radiol*. 2018;91(1087):20180132.

20. Badawy SZ, Etman A, Singh M, Murphy K, Mayelli T, Philadelphia M. Uterine artery embolization: the role in obstetrics and gynecology. *Clin Imaging*. 2001;25(4):288-295.

21. Singhal M, Gupta P, Sikka P, Khandelwal N. Uterine artery embolization following internal iliac arteries ligation in a case of post-partum hemorrhage: a technical challenge. *J Obstet Gynaecol India*. 2015;65(3):202-205.

22. Smith LA, Price N, Simonite V, Burns EE. Incidence of and risk factors for perineal trauma: a prospective observational study. *BMC Pregnancy Childbirth*. 2013;13:59.

23. Pergialiotis V, Vlachos D, Protopapas A, Pappa K, Vlachos G. Risk factors for severe perineal lacerations during childbirth. *Int J Gynaecol Obstet*. 2014;125(1):6-14.

24. Duncan A, Widekind CV. *Bleeding From the Lower Genital Tract*; 2012. Available at https://pdfs.semanticscholar.org/fdf3/636b6c264bb1f814ef986d12bd1d0be33d74.pdf?_ga=2.143732406.2045128397.1544387762-1542823851.1526926947. Accessed January 31, 2019.

25. Pelage JP, Le Dref O, Jacob D, Soyer P, Herbreteau D, Rymer R. Selective arterial embolization of the uterine arteries in the management of intractable post-partum hemorrhage. *Acta Obstet Gynecol Scand*. 1999;78(8):698-703.

26. Koganemaru M, Nonoshita M, Iwamoto R, et al. Endovascular management of intractable postpartum hemorrhage caused by vaginal laceration. *Cardiovasc Intervent Radiol*. 2016;39(8):1159-1164.

27. Eller AG, Bennett MA, Sharshiner M, et al. Maternal morbidity in cases of placenta accreta managed by a multidisciplinary care team compared with standard obstetric care. *Obstet Gynecol*. 2011;117(2 Pt 1):331-337.

28. Robinson BK, Grobman WA. Effectiveness of timing strategies for delivery of individuals with placenta previa and accreta. *Obstet Gynecol*. 2010;116(4):835-842.

29. Clark A, Farber MK, Sviggum H, Camann W. Cesarean delivery in the hybrid operating suite: a promising new location for high-risk obstetric procedures. *Anesth Analg*. 2013;117(5):1187-1189.

30. *Resources for Optimal Care of the Injured Patient*. 6th ed. Committee on Trauma, American College of Surgeons; 2014. Available at https://www.facs.org/~/media/files/quality%20programs/trauma/vrc%20resources/resources%20for%20optimal%20care.ashx. Accessed December 9, 2018.

31. Dubois J, Garel L, Grignon A, Lemay M, Leduc L. Placenta percreta: balloon occlusion and embolization of the internal iliac arteries to reduce intraoperative blood losses. *Am J Obstet Gynecol*. 1997;176(3):723-726.

32. Zwart JJ, Dijk PD, van Roosmalen J. Peripartum hysterectomy and arterial embolization for major obstetric hemorrhage: a 2-year nationwide cohort study in the Netherlands. *Am J Obstet Gynecol*. 2010;202(2):150.e1-150.e7.

33. Kirby JM, Kachura JR, Rajan DK, et al. Arterial embolization for primary postpartum hemorrhage. *J Vasc Interv Radiol*. 2009;20(8):1036-1045.

34. Pfizer GELFOAM® and GEL-FLOW NT. Available at https://www.pfizer.com/sites/default/files/products/uspi_gelfoam_plus.pdf. Accessed October 2019.

35. Waltman AC, Courey WR, Athanasoulis C, Baum S. Technique for left gastric artery catheterization. *Radiology*. 1973;109(3):732-734.
36. Broadwell SR, Ray CE. Transcatheter embolization in pelvic trauma. *Semin Intervent Radiol*. 2004;21(1):23-35.
37. Marso SP, Amin AP, House JA, et al. Association between use of bleeding avoidance strategies and risk of periprocedural bleeding among patients undergoing percutaneous coronary intervention. *J Am Med Assoc*. 2010;303(21):2156-2164.
38. Abando A, Hood D, Weaver F, Katz S. The use of the Angioseal device for femoral artery closure. *J Vasc Surg*. 2004;40(2):287-290.
39. Toor SS, Jaberi A, Macdonald DB, McInnes MD, Schweitzer ME, Rasuli P. Complication rates and effectiveness of uterine artery embolization in the treatment of symptomatic leiomyomas: a systematic review and meta-analysis. *Am J Roentgenol*. 2012;199(5):1153-1163.
40. Goldberg J, Pereira L, Berghella V. Pregnancy after uterine artery embolization. *Obstet Gynecol*. 2002;100(5 Pt 1):869-872.
41. Tan CH, Tay KH, Sheah K, et al. Perioperative endovascular internal iliac artery occlusion balloon placement in management of placenta accreta. *Am J Roentgenol*. 2007;189(5):1158-1163.
42. Cali G, Forlani F, Giambanco L, et al. Prophylactic use of intravascular balloon catheters in women with placenta accreta, increta and percreta. *Eur J Obstet Gynecol Reprod Biol*. 2014;179:36-41.
43. Ballas J, Hull AD, Saenz C, et al. Preoperative intravascular balloon catheters and surgical outcomes in pregnancies complicated by placenta accreta: a management paradox. *Am J Obstet Gynecol*. 2012;207(3):216.e1-216.e5.
44. Picel AC, Wolford B, Cochran RL, Ramos GA, Roberts AC. Prophylactic internal iliac artery occlusion balloon placement to reduce operative blood loss in patients with invasive placenta. *J Vasc Interv Radiol*. 2018;29(2):219-224.
45. Carnevale FC, Kondo MM, de Oliveira Sousa W Jr, et al. Perioperative temporary occlusion of the internal iliac arteries as prophylaxis in cesarean section at risk of hemorrhage in placenta accreta. *Cardiovasc Intervent Radiol*. 2011;34(4):758-764.
46. Panici PB, Anceschi M, Borgia ML, et al. Intraoperative aorta balloon occlusion: fertility preservation in patients with placenta previa accreta/increta. *J Matern Fetal Neonatal Med*. 2012;25(12):2512-2516.
47. Salim R, Chulski A, Romano S, Garmi G, Rudin M, Shalev E. Precesarean prophylactic balloon catheters for suspected placenta accreta: a randomized controlled trial. *Obstet Gynecol*. 2015;126(5):1022-1028.
48. Shrivastava V, Nageotte M, Major C, Haydon M, Wing D. Case-control comparison of cesarean hysterectomy with and without prophylactic placement of intravascular balloon catheters for placenta accreta. *Am J Obstet Gynecol*. 2007;197(4):402.e1-402.e5.
49. Blumenthal E, Rao R, Murphy A, et al. Pilot study of intra-aortic balloon occlusion to limit morbidity in patients with adherent placentation undergoing cesarean hysterectomy. *AJP Rep*. 2018;8(2):e57-e63.
50. Bodner LJ, Nosher JL, Gribbin C, Siegel RL, Beale S, Scorza W. Balloon-assisted occlusion of the internal iliac arteries in patients with placenta accreta/percreta. *Cardiovasc Intervent Radiol*. 2006;29(3):354-361.
51. Hughes CW. Use of an intra-aortic balloon catheter tamponade for controlling intra-abdominal hemorrhage in man. *Surgery*. 1954;36(1):65-68.
52. Zhu B, Yang K, Cai L. Discussion on the timing of balloon occlusion of the abdominal aorta during a caesarean section in patients with pernicious placenta previa complicated with placenta accreta. *Biomed Res Int*. 2017;2017:8604849.
53. Wu Q, Liu Z, Zhao X, et al. Outcome of pregnancies after balloon occlusion of the infrarenal abdominal aorta during caesarean in 230 patients with placenta praevia accreta. *Cardiovasc Intervent Radiol*. 2016;39(11):1573-1579.
54. Qiu Z, Hu J, Wu J, Chen L. Prophylactic temporary abdominal aorta balloon occlusion in women with placenta previa accretism during late gestation. *Medicine (Baltimore)*. 2017;96(46):e8681.
55. Luo F, Wu Z, Mei J, Yue J, Yu X, Xie L. Thrombosis after aortic balloon occlusion during cesarean delivery for abnormally invasive placenta. *Int J Obstet Anesth*. 2018;33:32-39.
56. Cui S, Zhi Y, Cheng G, Zhang K, Zhang L, Shen L. Retrospective analysis of placenta previa with abnormal placentation with and without prophylactic use of abdominal aorta balloon occlusion. *Int J Gynaecol Obstet*. 2017;137(3):265-270.
57. Stensaeth KH, Sovik E, Haig IN, Skomedal E, Jorgensen A. Fluoroscopy-free resuscitative endovascular balloon occlusion of the aorta (REBOA) for controlling life threatening postpartum hemorrhage. *PLoS One*. 2017;12(3):e0174520.

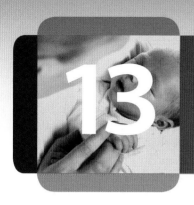

13 Operative Suite Prerequisites for Successful Outcomes

Guy I. Benrubi

INTRODUCTION

In the United States, if not worldwide, a cesarean delivery is the most commonly performed abdominal operation and except for cataract surgery, the most commonly performed procedure in medicine.[1] The estimates are that in 2018 there will be approximately 1,300,000 cesarean deliveries in the United States and 30 million worldwide. To put these numbers in perspective, the current estimate is that there is one cesarean section performed **every second** somewhere in the world.[2] There are two aspects of this procedure, which lead to a somewhat cavalier attitude toward the potential complications which may arise. As in the concept that "familiarity often breeds contempt," such a frequently performed operation is all too often taken for granted as being routine. The other influencing issue is that the procedure in its basic form is not complicated. In some ways, it is not an operation at all, but essentially an *open and close* process. In the standard case, it is a matter of entering several layers—skin, subcutaneous fat, fascia, peritoneum, uterus—removing an infant without requiring any *surgical maneuvers*, and then closing all the layers in proper sequence. It does not require any operative manipulations, such as removing a gall bladder or an appendix or a uterus, once the layers are open.

In the operative suite, the instrumentation required is minimal, and all too frequently, the C-section tray is significantly sparser than a hysterectomy tray in the same hospital. Many, if not most, hospitals have a hysterectomy tray readily available in Labor and Delivery, but this does not hold true for all obstetric operative suites around the country.

The most important prerequisite for the safe and efficacious performance of any surgical procedure or intervention is proper preparation. Obvious components include an understanding of the indications for the procedure, the goals of therapy, the potential pitfalls and complications which may be encountered during the procedure, and the immediate postprocedure and long-term consequences.[3] Inherent in preparation is having the proper tools to accomplish the tasks, which also implies the knowledge and training with the use of such tools. Expanding on the old adage, "if your only tool is a hammer, everything appears like a nail" we can say, "if the only tool with which you are comfortable using is a hammer, then everything to you will look like a nail."

OPERATING ROOM FACILITY

The single most important approach in adequately preparing the operating suite for the *difficult cesarean section* is to first and foremost realize that the team is not dealing with the standard *open-and-close* cesarean section, but a pelvic and an abdominal operation which could potentially be as complex as a pelvic exenteration or an abdominal/perineal resection. Whatever mental and resource preparations are required for those complex surgical operations, the same preparation is required for the difficult cesarean delivery.

The operating room space should be adequate space to accommodate the multimember team. If an accreta is known beforehand, the procedure should probably be scheduled in a main OR suite. The operating tables should be adequate to accommodate possibly multiple "scrubbed" surgeons and technicians, and patients with a high body mass index (BMI). Lighting is critical, and personal head lamps may be necessary. Communication systems with potential intraoperative consultants should be in working order. The anesthesia team should be comfortable with management of rapid fluid changes, possible requirement of massive transfusion therapy, the management of central monitoring, and prolonged anesthesia times, as a minimum.

INSTRUMENTS AND EQUIPMENT

Below is a list of equipment and instruments required in a cesarean tray. This standard cesarean tray is more than adequate to enable the obstetrician to perform the procedure safely and expeditiously. In most cesarean delivery procedures, most of these instruments would be superfluous. However, in a difficult case, this list would be inadequate and needs expansion to include other instruments and equipment as described below (Figure 13-1).

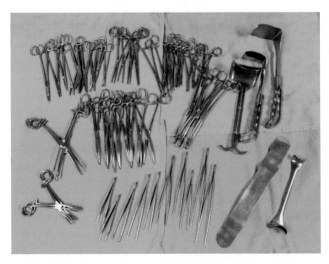

FIGURE 13-1 A standard C-section tray may not have sufficient instruments for complicated cesarean delivery.

STANDARD CESAREAN-SECTION TRAY

- Mosquito Crvd
- Mosquito Str
- Oschner Str
- Allis Tissue Forceps
- Needle Holders
- Mayo Scissor Crvd
- Metzenbaum Scissor Str/Crvd
- Bandage Scissor
- Babcock Tissue Forcep
- Tenaculum Forcep
- Sponge Forcep
- Towel Clamp
- Richardson Retractor
- Center Blade Retractor
- #3 Knife Handle
- Dressing Forcep
- Tissue Forcep
- Adson Tissue Forcep
- Russian Forcep

To the above list, the following must be added with description of when and why they are needed. The first components would be essentially the same as those found in a standard hysterectomy tray (Figure 13-2).

HYSTERECTOMY TRAY

- Scalpel Handle #3L
- Mayo Dissecting Scissors Cvd 6 3/4″
- Rochester-Ochsner Forceps Cvd 8″
- Rochester-Ochsner Forceps Str 8″
- Russian Tissue Forceps
- Heaney Needle Holder
- Allis Tissue Forceps 5 × 6 Teeth 9 1/2″
- DeBakey Tissue Forceps
- Mixter Right Angle Forceps
- Metzenbaum Scissors Cvd
- Deaver Retractor 1″ × 9″
- Deaver Retractor 1″ × 12″
- Deaver Retractor 1 1/2″ × 12″
- Schnidt Hemostat Cvd
- Foerster Sponge Forceps Str 9 1/2″
- Heaney Clamp
- Heaney-Ballantine Clamp Str
- Heaney-Ballantine Clamp Cvd

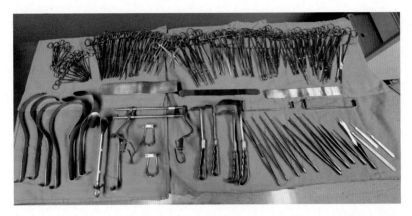

FIGURE 13-2 Instrument tray typically used in oncologic gynecologic surgery. These instruments are very frequently necessary in difficult cesarean sections. Radical hysterectomy tray has additional instruments which may be necessary for complicated cesarean deliveries.

Types of Retractors

For exposure there are two major types of retractors. There are fixed retractors and nonfixed retractors.

Fixed Retractors

The fixed retractors are the Bookwalter and the Omni (Figure 13-3). Both have a fixed arm, which attaches to the operating table. This allows for excellent exposure without operator or assistant fatigue. The Bookwalter has a ring to which various types of retractor blades can be attached. The Omni does not have a fixed ring and thus may be of additional help in obese patients, as the extent of lateral retraction is not limited by the width of the ring as with the Bookwalter.

Nonfixed Retractors

The nonfixed retractors include the Balfour and the O'Connor-O'Sullivan (Figure 13-4). They are easy to use and easily deployed, and most gynecologists are familiar with these as they are frequently used for open hysterectomies in nonobese patients. As the fixed retractors require some facility with their deployment, but well worth the extra time at the beginning of the case, surgeons attempting the difficult cesarean delivery, such as with an accreta, or an obese patient should be comfortable with the use of fixed retractors.

Additional Instruments Needed From the Gynecology/ Oncology Tray

In addition to the hysterectomy tray and the retractors, the surgeon performing a difficult cesarean, such as with known accreta, obese patient, or in a case of a fourth-repeated (*four-peat*) or higher procedure, should have the following instruments which are normally found in a gynecology/oncology tray. The obstetrician should be comfortable using these instruments or have ready access to a surgeon who is. In

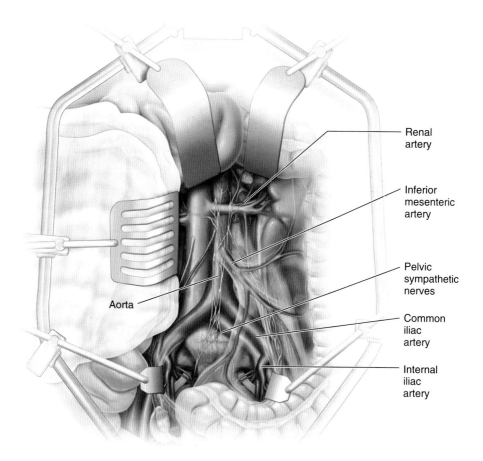

Renal artery

Inferior mesenteric artery

Pelvic sympathetic nerves

Common iliac artery

Internal iliac artery

Aorta

FIGURE 13-3 Operative exposure. The Omni-Tract or similar self-retaining retractor system permits the wide exposure of the operative field necessary. Omni retractor showing ability to get maximum exposure. (With permission from Darling RC, Ozaki CK. Master Techniques in Surgery; Vascular Surgery: Arterial Procedures. © Lippincott Williams & Wilkins/Wolters Kluwer; 2015 [Figure 20-3].)

obese patients, as in deep pelvic procedures such as with percreta attachments to deep structures, long instruments are essential.

- Long instruments: long Mayo scissors, long Metzenbaum scissors, long DeBakey forceps, long clamps, long sponge/ring clamps, long Babcocks etc. (Figure 13-5)
- Long wide Deaver retractors sometimes referred to as an *elephant Deaver*—at least 4 inches wide blade with a 12 inch handle (Figure 13-6).

Hemoclips

Hemoclips with both short and long clip appliers; these clips come in small medium and large, and all three sizes may become necessary. In deep pelvic situations, knot tying is difficult as well as fatiguing. Hemoclips come to the rescue.

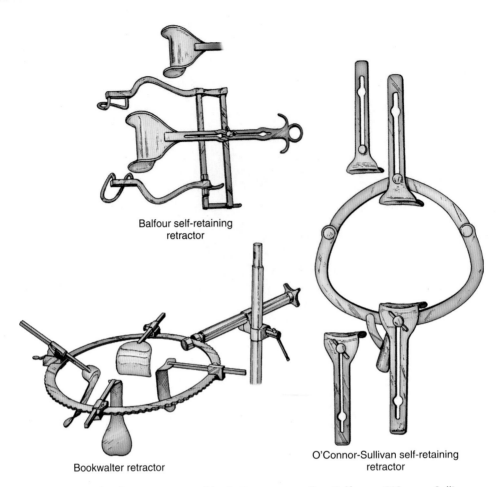

Balfour self-retaining retractor

Bookwalter retractor

O'Connor-Sullivan self-retaining retractor

FIGURE 13-4 Bookwalter retractor provides better exposure than Balfour or O'Connor-Sullivan self-retaining particularly in high BMI (body mass index) patients. (With permission from Handa VL, Van Le L. Te Linde's Operative Gynecology. 12th ed. © Lippincott Williams & Wilkins/Wolters Kluwer; 2019 [Figure 5-9]. Courtesy of Zinnanti Surgical, Santa Cruz, CA.)

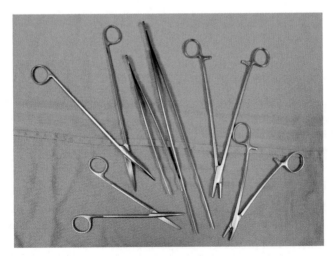

FIGURE 13-5 Long instruments are crucial in many difficult patients, particularly in high BMI (body mass index) patients.

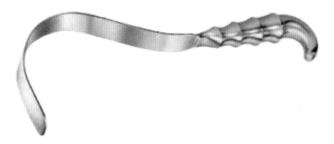

FIGURE 13-6 Deavers come in all sizes. The largest size (650 × 302) in sometimes called an "elephant Deaver" is crucial in high BMI (body mass index) patients. Please note the "comfort" handle. Accurate Surgical & Scientific Instruments Corporation (Westbury, NY).

Automated Stapling Devices (Figure 13-7)

Automated stapling devices are especially useful if adhesions are anticipated as well as potential risk for bowel injury. Though it is highly unlikely that a circular end-to-end anastomosis device will be needed (CEEA), a linear gastrointestinal device (GIA) and a thoracoabdominal device (TA) are frequently required. If there are extensive adhesions, especially omental, the ligate-divide-staple (LDS) instrument can be a significant time saver.

Suction Setups and Ring Forceps

As a minimum, two suction setups, with both pool and direct suction heads. Additional ring forceps should be available. They are excellent for temporary hemostasis in cut uterine surfaces.

Vascular Clamps (Figure 13-8)

Vascular clamps can be used to occlude major vessels without causing additional damage. They can be used to occlude the vessel above and below the injury so that the damage can be repaired. They also can be used to temporarily decrease blood flow, thus enabling the completion of a procedure and then restoring flow once the process is completed. Using a vascular clamp on the infundibulopelvic ligament to occlude the ovarian artery can be helpful. There are several vascular clamps on the market. The surgeon can decide the variety of her/his preference. In the author's experience, Bulldog clamps have been found very useful.

Intra-abdominal packs

Frequently in complicated cesarean deliveries, the procedure may have to be interrupted because of difficulty in obtaining hemostasis. This necessitates an abdominal packing of the bleeding area, usually in the deep pelvis, or the pelvic side wall, with the subsequent use of interventional radiology to identify and embolize the major source of bleeding. For packing in such situations Kerlix rolls have been found to be easily applied; they provide excellent absorptive surface and can be used for bulk pressure—can be tied end to end if necessary.

Additionally QuikClot rolls can be used.[4] QuikClot was developed by the military post the attacks on 9/11 and has been extensively used in Afghanistan and Iraq and

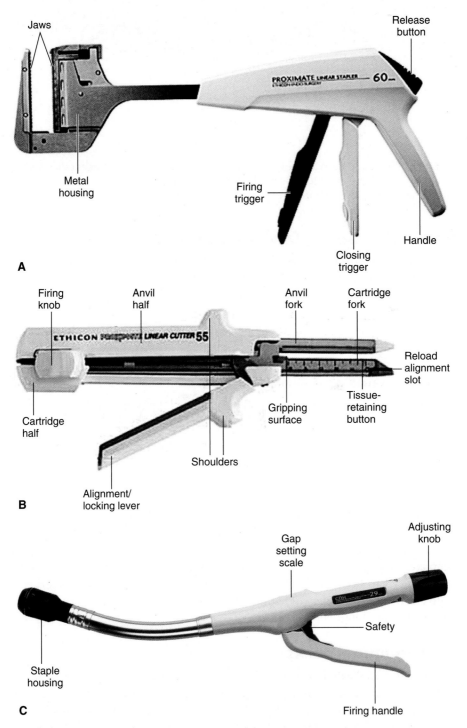

FIGURE 13-7 A-C. There are various staplers, disposable or multiuse. Shown here are circular end-to-end anastomosis device (CEEA), a linear gastrointestinal device (GIA), and a thoracoabdominal device (TA). (With permission from Berek JS, Hacker NF. Berek and Hacker's Gynecologic Oncology. 9th ed. © Lippincott Williams & Wilkins/Wolters Kluwer; 2014 [Figure 20-1].)

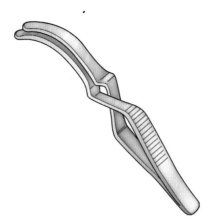

FIGURE 13-8 Bulldog vascular clamp can be very useful in temporary hemostasis by clamping the infundibulopelvic ligaments.

other combat situations. It is a kaolin-infused roll or gauze. Kaolin is a clay derivative, has no animal protein, and is well tolerated by tissues. It produces clotting by activating factor XII. Though the FDA has approved QuikClot (Figure 13-9) for external use only, there is now a body of literature that shows the product to be safe in internal tissues such as the vagina and intraperitonealy.[5] There has been extensive use of the product in intra-abdominal injuries in multiple Level I trauma centers. Both Kerlix and QuikClot have to be removed from the intra-abdominal sites, as they are not absorbable products. However, there is evidence that leaving them in place for up to 24 hours is safe.[6]

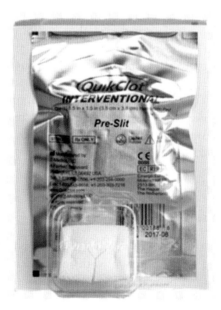

FIGURE 13.9 QuikClot product comes in multiple sizes. (From QuikClot.com, Z-Medica LLC Wallingford CT. Z-Medica.com. All rights reserved.)

Availability of Mass Transfusion Products

These "packs" and the standard guidelines are in use in Level I trauma centers, but should be readily available in cases where known accreta and percreta surgery is attempted. These packs contain packed cells, fresh-frozen plasma, platelets, and cryoprecipitate. The team in the OR should be in agreement as to the ratio of blood products that should be administered.

Tranexamic Acid

Tranexamic acid for intravenous administration should be available.[7,8] Tranexamic acid is an antifibrinolytic agent that can be given intravenously or orally. In a large, randomized trial, 1 g of intravenous tranexamic acid in the setting of postpartum hemorrhage, a significant reduction of mortality in the subgroup of death from obstetric hemorrhage was noted as compared to placebo. Tranexamic acid has also been shown to reduce obstetric blood loss when given prophylactically. Additionally, the risk of thrombosis was not different from controls. Furthermore, it seems that use within 3 hours from time of delivery has the best outcomes.

Cell Saver Capability

The use of the cell saver in obstetric cases was considered potentially unsafe because of amniotic fluid, as well as other concerns. During the peripartum period, cell salvage blood can be contaminated with bacteria, amniotic fluid, and fetal blood. Contamination by fetal blood is a definite concern because of possible antigen-antibody complexes that may form secondary to "Rh" type differences between the mother and the child. The potential to create an iatrogenic amniotic fluid embolus is the greatest fear that accompanies amniotic fluid contamination.

A 1991 article indicated that tissue factor is most likely involved in the disseminated intravascular coagulopathy that typically follows the acute embolic event of amniotic fluid embolus.[9-11] Tissue factor can be washed out during the cell saver process. A comprehensive article concluded that combining cell salvage washing and filtration produced a blood product that was similar to maternal blood. The exception to this conclusion was fetal hemoglobin contamination of maternal blood. Rhogam can be used to prevent isoimmunization. Support for the use of cell salvage in obstetric hemorrhage is now provided by over 400 reported cases in which blood contaminated with amniotic fluid has been washed and readministered without filtration. In addition, the American College of Obstetricians and Gynecologists have advocated the use of blood salvage in obstetrics, in their most recent Practice Bulletin on the subject.[12]

MULTIDISCIPLINARY TEAM

With proper preparation, the safety of the difficult cesarean delivery can be assured. But it requires a dedicated team approach, with several services, ancillary personnel, and hospital administration. A patient undergoing a difficult cesarean delivery may be as complicated as one with a challenging pelvic malignancy. In such patients a common sentiment is that "there is a need for a personalized, experienced, and well-organized multidisciplinary team management for every special patient to obtain best chance of cure." This sentiment should also be adopted when dealing with the patient about to undergo a difficult cesarean delivery.

Each member of the multidisciplinary team and their role is described in depth in Chapter 7: Intraoperative Management of Accreta, Percreta, and Increta.

Pelvic Surgeon

One of the most important prerequisites, if not the preeminent one, for the successful completion of the difficult cesarean delivery, is the availability of a pelvic surgeon who is comfortable with the potential involvement of pelvic structures which are not normally encountered in routine cesarean procedures. Increasingly academic health centers use a system of "senior surgeon" backup call. Frequently these individuals are gynecologic oncologists, but they do not have to be. What is important is the realization that the practice of a specialist in general obstetrics and gynecology is incredibly fragmented. This is a result of the tremendous increase in medical knowledge and technology which is over all an excellent outcome. However, the consequent result is that not every specialist in general obstetrics and gynecology can be an expert in all surgical eventualities. *Thus, appropriate intraoperative consultation must be available.*

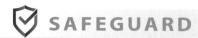 **SAFEGUARD**

Not every specialist in general obstetrics and gynecology can be an expert in all surgical eventualities. *Thus, appropriate intraoperative consultation must be available.*

First and foremost, the senior surgeon must be comfortable in operating in an *open abdomen*. Many pelvic surgeons are comfortable only with robotic or laparoscopic procedures. Increasingly labor and delivery suits are being managed by "laborists" and "nocturnalists," which is an excellent safety feature for management of labor, but there may be a possible lack of experience with complex surgical procedures.

The senior surgeon must also be comfortable with the anatomy and the handling of tissues in the retroperitoneal space. Many pelvic surgeons have essentially lived their whole surgical lives above the peritoneal reflection and medial to the lateral leaves of the peritoneum. Especially in situations of abnormal placentation and adhesions secondary to multiple procedures, the knowledge of anatomy of the para rectal, para vesical, and obturator spaces can be critical. The knowledge of the course of the ureter and its relation to retroperitoneal blood vessels is obligatory. Nerve supply of major organs and muscles must be taken into consideration.

The senior pelvic surgeon must be sufficiently comfortable with catastrophic intraoperative situations in order to maintain her or his "sangfroid". She or he must be familiar with extraordinary measures such as *fist compression of the aorta* and *fearless clamping* using instruments such as Ring forceps or Masterson clamps.

One of the fathers of gynecologic oncology used the following saying with his trainees: "It is not your blood, and remember that you did not give her the cancer." He thus indelibly etched in their minds that despite adverse intraoperative events, the surgeon needs to maintain composure, establish control of the situation, and take care of the patient.

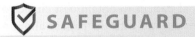 SAFEGUARD

It is more safe practice that a *four-peat* or higher section not be performed unless a backup senior surgeon is available.

As the number of repeat cesarean sections increases, the chances for major complications also rise. Most studies point to a marked increase in complications with the fourth-repeat cesarean section, especially if one of the previous sections had been done for a placenta previa.[13] It is a safe practice that a *four-peat* or higher section not be performed unless a backup senior surgeon is available.

Interventional Radiologist

Lastly, although this is a subject addressed in detail in Chapter 12: Role of Interventional Radiology in the Management of the Difficult Cesarean Delivery, emphasis must be given to the critical role of interventional radiology. Any busy obstetric service, especially those catering to a demographic population with a 50% or higher obesity rate (essentially inner city safety-net hospitals) must have an interventional radiology service readily available. The most common preventable cause of maternal mortality is obstetric hemorrhage.[12] Thus interventional radiology services are critically important in preventing many of these deaths.

REFERENCES

1. Cesarean Delivery Rate. Available at www.cdc.gov/nchs/pressroom/sosmap/cesarean-births/cesareans.htm. Accessed 12/2018.
2. Betran A, Jianfeng Y, Moller A, Zhang J, Gulmezoglu A, Torloni M. The increasing trend in caesarean section rates: global, regional, and national estimates: 1990-2014. *PLoS One*. 2016;11(2):e0148343.
3. ACOG Committee Opinion #750. *Obstet Gynecol*. 2018;132(3):e120-e130.
4. Gegel BT, Austin PN, Johnson AD. An evidence-based review of the use of a combat gauge (QuikClot™) for hemorrhage control. *Am Assoc Nurse Anesth J*. 2013;81(6):453-458.
5. Choron RL, Hazelton JP, Hunter K, et al. Intra-abdominal packing with laparotomy pads and QuickClot during damage control laparotomy: a safety analysis. *Injury*. 2017;48(1):158-164.
6. Vilardo N, Feinberg J, Black J, Ratner E. The use of QuikClot combat gauge in cervical and vaginal hemorrhage. *Gynecol Oncol Rep*. 2017;21:114-116.
7. Novikova N, Hofmeyr GJ, Cluver C. Tranexamic acid for preventing postpartum haemorrhage. *Cochrane Database Syst Rev*. 2015;(6):CD007872.
8. Simonazzi G, Bisulli M, Saccone G, Moro E, Marshall A, Berghella V. Tranexamic acid for preventing postpartum blood loss after cesarean delivery: a systematic review and meta-analysis of randomized controlled trials. *Acta Obstet Gynecol Scand*. 2016;95:28-37.
9. Waters JH, Biscotti C, Potter PS, Phillipson E. Amniotic fluid removal during cell salvage in the cesarean section patient. *Anesthesiology*. 2000;92:1531-1536.
10. Goucher H, Wong CA, Patel SK, Toledo P. Cell salvage in obstetrics. *Anesth Analg*. 2015;121:465-468.
11. Liumbruno GM, Liumbruno C, Rafanelli D. Intraoperative cell salvage in obstetrics: is it a real therapeutic option? *Transfusion*. 2011;51:2244-2256.
12. ACOG Practice Bulletin #183 October 2017. Available at www.acog.org/clinical-guidance-and-publications/Practice-Bulletins. Accessed February 10, 2019.
13. Resnik R, Silver R. Management of the Placenta Accreta Spectrum (Placenta Accreta, Increta, and Percreta). Available at http://www.uptodate.com/content/2018. Accessed February 10, 2019.

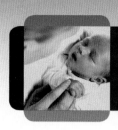

INDEX

Note: Page numbers followed by "f" indicate figures and "t" indicates tables.